Patient Management in the Telemetry/Cardiac Step Down Unit
A Case-Based Approach

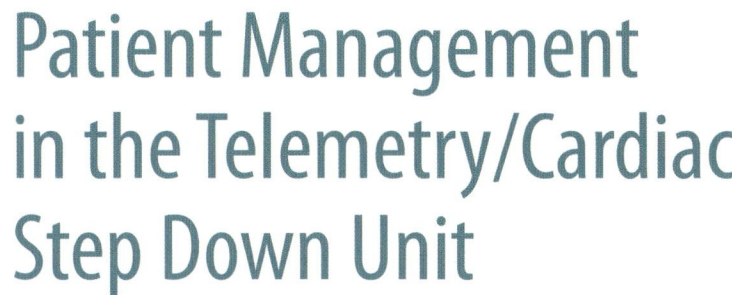

Patient Management in the Telemetry/Cardiac Step Down Unit

A Case-Based Approach

Editors

Muhammad Saad, MD
Department of Internal Medicine
BronxCare Hospital Center
Bronx, New York

Manoj Bhandari, MD
Department of Cardiology
BronxCare Hospital Center
Bronx, New York

Timothy J. Vittorio, MS, MD
Department of Cardiology
BronxCare Hospital Center
Bronx, New York

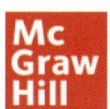

New York   Chicago   San Francisco   Athens   London   Madrid   Mexico City
Milan   New Delhi   Singapore   Sydney   Toronto

Patient Management in the Telemetry/Cardiac Step Down Unit: A Case-Based Approach

Copyright © 2020 by McGraw-Hill Education. All rights reserved. Printed in China.
Except as permitted under the United States Copyright Act of 1976, no part of this
publication may be reproduced or distributed in any form or by any means, or stored in a
data base or retrieval system, without the prior written permission of the publisher.

1 2 3 4 5 6 7 8 9   DSS   24 23 22 21 20 19

ISBN 978-1-260-45699-8
MHID 1-260-45699-4

This book was set in Minion Pro by Cenveo® Publisher Services.
The editors were Karen Edmonson and Christie Naglieri.
The production supervisor was Catherine Saggese
The text designer was Mary McKeon.
The index was prepared by Cenveo Publisher Services.
Project management was provided by Sarika Gupta, Cenveo Publisher Services.

This book is printed on acid-free paper.

Library of Congress Control Number:2019947604
Library of CongressUS Programs, Law, and Literature DivisionCataloging in Publication
Program101 Independence Avenue, S.E.Washington, DC 20540-4283

McGraw-Hill books are available at special quantity discounts to use as premiums and sales promotions,
or for use in corporate training programs. To contact a representative visit the Contact Us pages at
www.mhprofessional.com.

Acknowledgments

We would like to extend our gratitude to the following colleagues for their continuous support and encouragement during the writing of this book.

Dr. Sridhar Chilimuri, MD, FACG
Chairman, Department of Internal Medicine
BronxCare Hospital Center

Dr. Jonathan. N. Bella, MD, FACC, FASE, FAHA
Chief, Division of Cardiovascular Medicine
BronxCare Hospital Center

Dr. Muhammad Adrish, MD, FCCP
Attending Physician, Department of Pulmonary Medicine
BronxCare Hospital Center

Additionally, we are indebted to our families who allowed us time away to complete this endeavor.

Contents

Contributors

Fareeha S. Alavi, MD
Resident
Department of Internal Medicine
BronxCare Hospital Center
Bronx, New York

Nisha Ali, MD
Resident
Department of Internal Medicine
BronxCare Hospital Center
Bronx, New York

Muhammad Ameen, MBBS, MD
Attending Physician
Department of Internal Medicine
BronxCare Health System
Bronx, New York

Manoj Bhandari, MD
Attending Physician
Department of Cardiology
BronxCare Hospital Center
Bronx, New York

Gayathri Kamalakkannan, MD
Cardiologist
Department of Internal Medicine
BronxCare Hospital Center
Bronx, New York

Nikhitha Mantri, MD
Resident
Department of Internal Medicine
BronxCare Health System
New York, New York

Jeirym Miranda, MD
Resident
Department of Medicine
BronxCare Health System
Bronx, New York

Marin Nicu, MD
Attending Physician
Department of Cardiology
BronxCare Health System
Bronx, New York

Vincent Setiawan Prawoko, MD
Internal Medicine Resident
Department of Medicine
BronxCare Health System
Bronx, New York

Ayyadurai Puvanalingam, MD
Cardiology Fellow
Department of Cardiology
BronxCare Health System
New York, New York

Swathi Roy, MD
Resident
Department of Internal Medicine
BronxCare Hospital Center
Bronx, New York

Muhammad Saad, MD
Attending Physician
Department of Internal Medicine
BronxCare Hospital Center
Bronx, New York

Niel N. Shah, MD
Resident
Department of Internal Medicine
BronxCare Hospital Center
Bronx, New York

Timothy J. Vittorio, MS, MD
Department of Cardiology
BronxCare Hospital Center
Bronx, New York

Preface

This first edition of our textbook *Patient Management in the Telemetry/Cardiac Step Down Unit: A Case-Based Approach* was developed as a unique and practical means to assist physicians-in-training and other medical providers including nurse practitioners and physician assistants who work on a busy telemetry floor. We constructed the text as user friendly as possible by utilizing a personal conversation style.

This book is essentially a user's manual to assist the medical provider in making good clinical judgment quickly. The book is broken down into chapters based on common, genuine clinical cases with a proposed approach for each case.

To help orient the reader and to prevent the medical provider from excessive details, we added key points at the end of each case highlighting the major points throughout the clinical content with the goal of allowing an easy and quick review.

It is our hope that this book will serve as an effective teaching tool in learning telemetry medicine.

Muhammad Saad, MD
Manoj Bhandari, MD
Timothy J. Vittorio, MS, MD

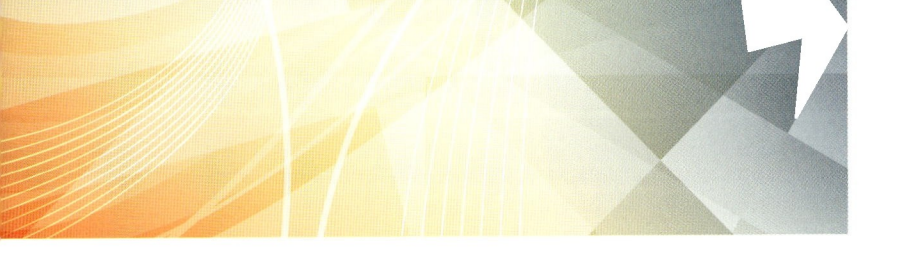

10 Real Cases on Acute Coronary Syndrome: Diagnosis, Management, and Follow-Up

Nisha Ali • Timothy J. Vittorio

CASE 1

Diagnostic Evaluation of Chest Pain

A 65-year-old man presented to the emergency department with a complaint of left-sided chest pain radiating to his left arm. There were no alleviating factors. His past medical history included hypertension, uncontrolled diabetes mellitus, and hyperlipidemia. He denied any toxic habits. His baseline exercise tolerance is 2 city blocks limited by fatigue. Upon presentation, vital signs were stable and the physical examination was unremarkable. The chest pain was partially relieved by sublingual nitroglycerin. The 12-lead ECG showed non-specific T-wave inversions in the inferolateral leads. He was administered aspirin, and the chest pain resolved shortly thereafter. Subsequently, he was admitted to the telemetry floor for further evaluation and observation. His serial cardiac biomarkers were negative. He did not have any recurrent chest pain and remained hemodynamically stable throughout the hospital stay. How would you manage this case?

Case Review

In this clinical scenario, the patient does not fit the complete picture of anginal symptoms. However, the key here is the presence of risk factors and subtle 12-lead ECG changes, which place him at an elevated risk for coronary artery disease. He can be further evaluated by stress testing for risk stratification.

Case Discussion

Angina consists of retrosternal chest pain increased by activity or emotional stress and generally relieved by rest or administration of nitroglycerin. The evaluation of chest pain begins with a thorough history and physical examination to delineate the etiology. The list of differential diagnoses is vast, and a detailed review of systems about pertinent diagnoses can narrow down the list. The presence of comorbid conditions and risk factors might hint toward a diagnosis of coronary artery disease. Both serial 12-lead ECG and highly sensitive cardiac troponin T testing should be performed before excluding ongoing ischemic coronary artery disease. Prior to stress testing, the patient should be chest pain free for 24 hours, without dynamic 12-lead ECG changes, and the highly sensitive cardiac troponin T level should be negative or trending downward.

The differential diagnosis of chest pain includes the following:

- Coronary artery disease
- Aortic dissection
- Pericarditis
- Pneumonia
- Pulmonary embolism
- Costochondritis/rib fracture
- Peptic ulcer disease
- Acute cholecystitis
- Cervical radiculopathy
- Herpes zoster
- Anxiety disorder

Key Points

- Chest pain should be classified as anginal or nonanginal based on the history.
- Anginal symptoms can be considered in the setting of risk factors and should be evaluated by an appropriate stress modality if the symptoms are vague.
- Serial 12-lead ECG and highly sensitive cardiac troponin T should be performed to exclude ongoing ischemic coronary artery disease before stress testing is performed.

CASE 2

Diagnosis of Acute Coronary Syndrome

A 56-year-old obese man presented to the emergency department with a complaint of central chest pain awakening him from sleep. He has a past medical history of hypertension and bronchial asthma. In addition, he is an active smoker and works full time as an office secretary. He self-administered acetaminophen, but it did not alleviate the discomfort. Upon arrival, he continued to have chest pain, which was not relieved by nitroglycerin. He appeared to be in mild distress; otherwise, the vital signs and physical examination were unremarkable. The 12-lead ECG showed ST-segment depressions in the anterior and lateral precordial leads (as shown in Figure 1.2.1). Treatment with aspirin, clopidogrel, and an unfractionated heparin infusion was begun. The highly sensitive cardiac troponin T level was elevated. Subsequently, he was admitted to the telemetry unit for further care, including a discussion about cardiac catheterization. The chest pain improved, and his decision was to defer an invasive strategy. The 12-lead ECG changes resolved, and the highly sensitive cardiac troponin T level trended downward. How would you manage this case further?

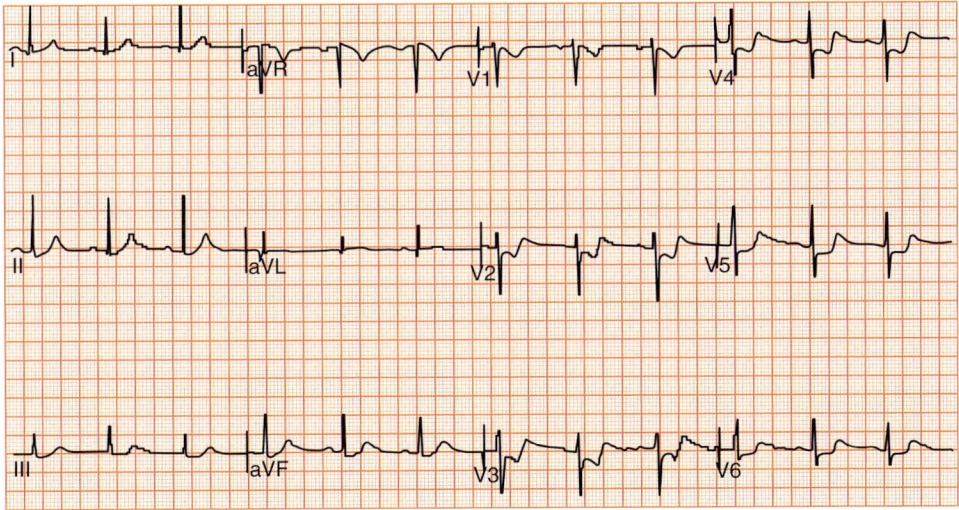

Figure 1.2.1 ST depression in inferio-lateral leads.

Case Review

Acute coronary syndrome consists of ST-segment elevation myocardial infarction (STEMI), non–ST-segment myocardial infarction (NSTEMI), and unstable angina (UA). In this clinical scenario, the patient was diagnosed with NSTEMI based on the clinical criteria of the 12-lead ECG changes and elevated highly sensitive cardiac troponin T level. The Thrombolysis in Myocardial Infarction (TIMI) risk score can be used to guide management (Table 1.2.1). A TIMI risk score of 3 is considered intermediate, and hence, a conservative strategy can be adopted, instead of an invasive strategy.

TABLE 1.2.1 Thrombolysis in Myocardial Infarction (TIMI) Score		
	Score	**Incidence of Mortality (%)**
Age ≥65 years	1	4.7
≥3 coronary artery disease risk factors	2	8.3
Prior coronary stenosis >50%	3	13
Presence of ST- segment deviation	4	20
≥2 episodes of angina within 24 hours	5	26
Elevated cardiac biomarkers	6	41
Prior use of aspirin in past 7 days	7	41

Total possible TIMI score is 7 points: a score of 1 to 2 is low risk; a score of 3 to 4 is intermediate risk; and a score of 4 to 7 is high risk.

Case Discussion

NSTEMI/UA may present as a new-onset or worsening of anginal symptoms with 12-lead ECG changes such as ST-segment depression, transient ST-segment elevation, or dynamic T-wave inversions with the presence of cardiac biomarkers (NSTEMI) or with absent cardiac biomarkers (UA) (Table 1.2.2). Plaque rupture, thrombus formation, and vasospasm can be the underlying mechanisms of occurrence.

Clinical Symptoms

Ongoing chest pain, heart failure symptoms, and syncope are signs of potentially worse outcomes.

Management

Initial management consists of nitrates, dual antiplatelet agents, anticoagulation, β-adrenergic blockers, and angiotensin-converting enzyme inhibitors (in the presence of left ventricular dysfunction). High-intensity 3-hydroxy-3-methylglutaryl–coenzyme A (HMG-CoA) reductase inhibitors (statins) should be initiated early during the hospital course. Patients with active symptoms and hemodynamic instability should be considered for early invasive therapy with cardiac catheterization. The TIMI risk score and/or Global Registry of Acute Coronary Events (GRACE) score can be used to guide both prognosis and management. Low- or intermediate-risk patients can be managed with optimal medical therapy. Stress testing should be performed before discharge or within 72 hours. High-risk candidates

TABLE 1.2.2 Diagnostic Algorithm for Acute Coronary Syndrome	
ST-segment elevation myocardial infarction	Angina and ST-segment elevation with positive troponin
Non–ST-segment elevation myocardial infarction	Angina, ST-segment deviation, T-wave inversion, and positive troponin
Unstable angina	New or worsening angina, ST-segment nonspecific changes, and negative troponin

should go for early invasive therapy. For the conservative strategy, a patient continuing to have symptoms or high risk of adverse events should undergo an invasive strategy. Low-risk candidates or patients with active chest pain with low probability of coronary artery disease can be managed with medical therapy.

Key Points

- Clinical symptoms, 12-lead ECG changes, and cardiac biomarkers are the cornerstone elements for the diagnosis of acute coronary syndrome. Serial 12-lead ECG and highly sensitive cardiac troponin T levels should be performed.
- The TIMI risk score can guide the management and prognosis.
- Dual antiplatelet agents, anticoagulation, and nitrates should be initiated regardless of the management strategy. Furthermore, β-adrenergic blockers should be started early in the hospital course.
- If a conservative strategy is adopted, then stress testing should be performed once the clinical symptoms have resolved.

CASE 3

Diagnosis of Anginal Variants

A 46-year-old man was evaluated by the emergency medical services with a complaint of chest pain. The on-site 12-lead ECG showed ST-segment elevation in the anterior precordial leads with ST-segment depression in the inferior leads (as shown in Figure 1.3.1). The local hospital ST-segment elevation myocardial infarction (STEMI) protocol was activated, and the patient was brought directly to the cardiac catheterization laboratory. The coronary artery anatomy demonstrated severe vasospasm, which improved with intracoronary nitroglycerin. The chest pain resolved, and he was admitted to the telemetry floor. He denied any medical conditions, and there was no family history of premature coronary artery disease. However, he is an active smoker and admitted intranasal cocaine use 1 night prior to the onset of his symptoms. Serial 12-lead ECG showed resolution of the ST-segment and T-wave changes. How would you manage this case?

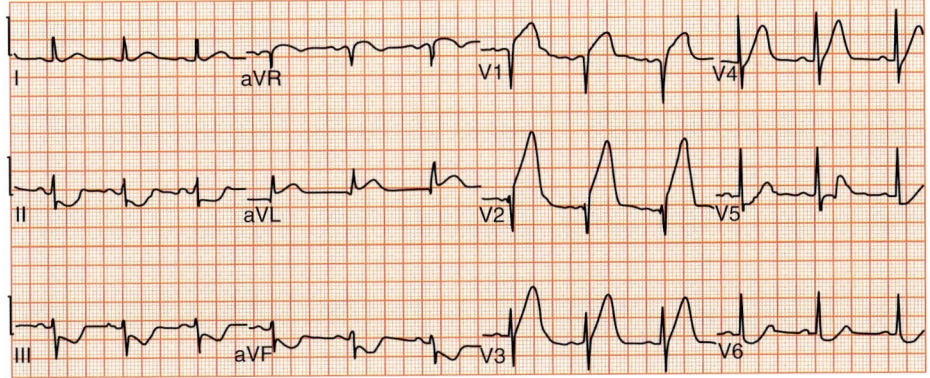

Figure 1.3.1 ST elevation in anterior leads with reciprocal changes.

Case Review

Prinzmetal or variant angina is in the differential diagnosis of acute coronary syndrome. Although the initial management is similar to that for acute coronary syndrome, it should be considered when the pretest probability of coronary artery disease is low. In this clinical scenario, the patient should be advised about smoking cessation and abstinence from recreational drug abuse.

Case Discussion

Prinzmetal or variant angina is defined as recurrent anginal symptoms that start at rest with transient 12-lead ECG changes and that are relieved by nitroglycerin. Decubitus angina with nocturnal awakening, syncope, and angina not associated with exertion are the components in the history. Cold exposure can be a trigger. The underlying mechanism is coronary vasospasm. The diagnosis can be made by clinical and angiographic evidence for vasospasm. Provocative testing is no longer suggested in the guidelines. The first-line treatment includes smoking cessation and avoidance of triggers. Vasodilators such as nitrates and calcium channel antagonists are used for symptomatic relief. β-Blockers should be avoided in these patients. Although it can be associated with sudden cardiac death due to the occurrence of malignant arrhythmias, long-term prognosis with early detection is generally favorable. The presence of underlying coronary artery disease should also be considered in the setting of traditional risk factors because mixed patterns can also be found.

Key Points

- Prinzmetal or variant angina is a differential for acute coronary syndrome.
- Angina at rest with transient 12-lead ECG changes relieved by nitrates and angiographic features of vasospasm are the key in diagnosis.
- Smoking cessation and use of vasodilators are the components of treatment. β-Blockers should be avoided.
- A mixed pattern with underlying coronary artery disease should also be considered.

CASE 4

Diagnosis of Musculoskeletal Chest Pain

A 35-year-old woman was evaluated in the emergency department for ongoing chest pain over the past week. She denied any shortness of breath, palpitation, nausea, vomiting, or pyrosis. She has no past medical or surgical history and is not receiving treatment with medication. There is no family history of coronary artery disease. The vital signs were stable. The cardiopulmonary examination revealed tenderness to palpation over the left parasternal region. The 12-lead ECG showed normal sinus rhythm, and chest radiography demonstrated no abnormalities. Cardiac biomarkers are pending in the chemistry laboratory. Pregnancy test was negative. What is the most likely diagnosis, and how would you manage this condition?

Case Review

In this clinical secnario, the young woman without risk factors for coronary artery disease should be evaluated for other causes of chest pain.

Case Discussion

Costochondritis, or Tietze syndrome (also called chondropathia tuberosa or costochon-dral junction syndrome), is an inflammation of the costochondral junctions of ribs of the chondrosternal joints. The exact cause of costochondritis is unknown. However, it can be caused by trauma, physical strain, arthritis, tumor in the costosternal region, and in some cases, infections.

Clinical Symptoms

Pain and tenderness usually occur on the sides of the sternum and are often worsened with cough, deep breathing, or strenuous physical activity.

Management

In most cases, a thorough history and physical examination are enough to consider the diagnosis. However, 12-lead ECG, chest radiography, and cardiac biomarkers must be per-formed to exclude other causes of chest pain.

Costochondritis usually resolves on its own or with rest. Patient with mild to moderate symptoms can be treated with nonsteroidal anti-inflammatory drugs (NSAIDs), analge-sics, or in some cases, tricyclic antidepressants, including amitriptyline and corticosteroid injections.

Key Points

- It is important to assess the pretest probability for the diagnosis before initiation of the workup. A consideration of risk factors for coronary artery disease is an important key to guide the approach.

CASE 5

Diagnosis of Stress Cardiomyopathy

A 58-year-old postmenopausal woman presented to the emergency department with com-plaints of severe substernal chest pain for the past 2 hours that was nonradiating and asso-ciated with shortness breath. The chest pain started suddenly when she was talking with her son on the phone. The pain was not relieved by aspirin. Recently, she moved from Florida to New York and has been living a stressful lifestyle to meet her needs. Her medical history includes well-controlled hypertension, diabetes mellitus, and depression. On arrival, the patient appeared in mild distress, but otherwise, her vital signs were stable. The cardio-pulmonary examination showed no abnormality. The 12-lead ECG showed ST-segment elevation in the anterior precordial leads V_1 to V_3 with diffuse T-wave inversions. The lab-oratory results revealed an elevated highly sensitive cardiac troponin level. The patient was administered aspirin, clopidogrel, and an unfractionated heparin infusion. Emergent left cardiac catheterization showed patent coronary artery anatomy. The left ventricular angio-gram showed basal left ventricular hyperkinesis with a severe left ventricular apical systolic wall motion abnormality. How would you approach this case?

Case Review

Stress-induced or takotsubo cardiomyopathy, also known as neurogenic stunned myocardium or broken heart syndrome, is a type of nonischemic cardiomyopathy that is characterized by transient left ventricular systolic dysfunction precipitated by intense acute emotional or physical stress. In this clinical scenario, although the woman has traditional risk factors for coronary artery disease, the fact that she has been experiencing emotional stress is the clue. The clinical presentation is classic for acute myocardial infarction, and therefore, the algorithm of its diagnosis follows the management for acute coronary syndrome.

Case Discussion

Takotsubo cardiomyopathy mimics acute coronary syndrome and is accompanied by reversible left ventricular apical ballooning. The exact pathophysiology of stress-induced cardiomyopathy is unclear. Postulated mechanisms include catecholamine-induced myocyte injury, transient coronary artery vasospasm, and microvascular dysfunction. The condition is also observed in patients with septic shock patients and acute cerebrovascular accident.

Clinical Symptoms

Symptoms include severe substernal chest pain, dyspnea, and syncope.

Management

Stress cardiomyopathy mimics acute myocardial infarction, with 12-lead ECG changes (ST-segment elevation, T-wave inversion, and QTc prolongation) and elevated cardiac biomarkers. Wall motion abnormalities are typically regional and extend beyond a single epicardial coronary artery distribution. The diagnosis is confirmed by left cardiac catheterization, which shows patent coronary artery anatomy with an akinetic or hypokinetic left ventricular apex leading to systolic left ventricular apical ballooning.

Treatment includes supportive care until left ventricular function is recovered. Medical therapy consists of β-adrenergic blockers and angiotensin-converting enzyme inhibitors. Short-term prognosis is generally favorable, but data on long-term outcomes are limited.

Key Points

- Takotsubo cardiomyopathy should be considered in the differential diagnosis of acute myocardial infarction and/or acute coronary syndrome.
- The diagnostic algorithm consists of a thorough history and physical examination with a typical pattern seen on both the transthoracic echocardiogram and left ventriculography.
- Conservative treatment is used with optimum outcome.

CASE 6

Diagnosis of Acute Pulmonary Embolism

A 32-year-old woman was evaluated in the emergency department for chest pain that started 3 hours ago. The chest pain worsened with deep inspiration and was associated with dyspnea. There were no other medical comorbid conditions. The past surgical history included a cesarean section. The only prescription medications included oral contraceptive pills (OCPs). On physical examination, the patient appeared tachypneic and in mild distress. The blood pressure was 100/60 mm Hg, pulse rate was 130 bpm, and respiratory rate was 26 breaths/min. The 12-lead ECG showed sinus tachycardia without ST-T–wave changes. The laboratory data revealed elevated levels of highly sensitive cardiac troponin and D-dimer. The patient received aspirin and nitroglycerin without relief of symptoms. What is the most likely cause of the ongoing chest pain?

Case Review

Venous thromboembolism should be considered in the evaluation for chest pain when risk factors for coronary artery disease are absent. In this clinical scenario, with the exception of sinus tachycardia, despite the absence of 12-lead ECG changes, a young woman with OCP use and elevated D-dimer points toward a diagnosis of acute pulmonary embolism.

Case Discussion

Pulmonary embolism (PE) is a blockage of 1 of the pulmonary arteries. The cause is usually a blood clot in the leg that breaks loose and travels through the bloodstream to the lung.

Risk Factors

- Prolonged immobilization, mainly after surgery or travel requiring sitting for long periods
- Estrogen-containing hormonal contraception
- Pregnancy
- Cancer
- Genetic thrombophilia (factor V Leiden, prothrombin mutation, protein C deficiency, protein S deficiency, antithrombin III deficiency, hyperhomocysteinemia)
- Acquired thrombophilia such as antiphospholipid syndrome

Clinical Symptoms

Symptoms include pleuritic chest pain, cough, dizziness, dyspnea, hemoptysis, and syncope. In some cases, sudden cardiac death may occur.

Evaluation

Evaluation of PE should include etiology in order to identify the PE as provoked or unprovoked, which can assist in further workup and help guide duration of treatment.

Twelve-Lead ECG. Sinus tachycardia is seen in most cases. Other findings include right axis deviation, incomplete or complete right bundle branch block with evidence for right heart strain, deep S wave in lead I, and Q-wave and T-wave inversion in lead III (S1Q3T3 pattern).

Laboratory Values. Values include elevated highly sensitive cardiac troponin T, B-type natriuretic peptide (more prognostic than diagnostic), and D-dimer levels.

Chest Radiography. Normal versus pleural effusion or atelectasis. A Hampton hump and the Palla and Westermark signs are rare but, when present, should raise the suspicion for acute PE.

A Hampton hump sign is a wedge-shaped opacification abutting the pleura in the periphery of the affected lung field. A Westermark sign is an area of focal oligemia distal to the hypoperfused lung field. The Palla sign is a dilated and/or enlarged right descending pulmonary artery.

Transthoracic Echocardiography. McConnell sign is the classic finding of mid-free right ventricular wall akinesis with normal motion of the right ventricular apex. Normal cardiac function and structure on echocardiogram suggest good prognosis.

Venous Doppler Duplex Ultrasound of the Lower Extremities. This test is performed to diagnose deep venous thrombosis.

Wells Score Pretest Probability. The Wells score is the most commonly used method to predict clinical probability of a PE. The Wells score consists of the following:

- Clinically suspected deep venous thrombosis = 3.0 points
- Alternative diagnosis is less likely than acute PE = 3.0 points
- Tachycardia (heart rate >100 bpm) = 1.5 points
- Immobilization (≥3 days) or surgery in previous 4 weeks = 1.5 points
- Prior history of deep venous thrombosis or acute PE = 1.5 points
- Hemoptysis = 1.0 point
- Malignancy (treatment within past 6 months) = 1.0 point

A score of <2 indicates low probability; a score of 2 to 6 indicates intermediate probability, and score of >6 indicates high probability.

In low-probability cases, D-dimer is useful. If D-dimer is negative, then acute PE can be excluded. In intermediate-probability cases, if the D-dimer is negative, then acute PE is excluded. If the D-dimer is >500 ng/mL, then chest CT angiography or a ventilation/perfusion (V/Q) scan should be performed. In high-probability cases, the patient should receive anticoagulation and more definitive studies such as chest CT angiography or V/Q scan.

Management

Anticoagulation therapy is the mainstay of treatment. It includes low-molecular-weight heparin and unfractionated heparin, which can later be changed to warfarin or one of the newer direct oral anticoagulants (apixaban, dabigatran, or rivaroxaban). Provoked and first unprovoked PE require 3 months of treatment. Supportive treatment such as oxygen or analgesia may be required.

In patients who are hemodynamically unstable, thrombolysis or mechanical thrombectomy may be required.

Key Points

- PE presents with pleuritic chest pain along with dyspnea and hemoptysis.
- Pretest probability can be assessed using the Wells score: D-dimer can be used to exclude acute PE if the clinical suspicion is low, but chest CT angiography is required in highly suspected cases.
- Long-term anticoagulation with direct oral anticoagulants is the mainstay of treatment.

CASE 7

Diagnosis of Aortic Dissection

A 75-year-old man was evaluated in the emergency department for a complaint of sudden onset of chest pain that started 2 hours ago. The pain radiated toward his back and was described as tearing in nature. He denied any neurologic symptoms. The past medical history included uncontrolled hypertension and dyslipidemia. The medication regimen consisted of amlodipine and hydrochlorothiazide. Two weeks ago, however, he ran out of his prescriptions and has not taken any of his medications since. On physical examination, he appeared in mild distress. The vital signs showed a blood pressure of 220/105 mm Hg, pulse rate of 90 bpm, and respiratory rate of 20 breaths/min. The pulses were equal bilaterally. The cardiac examination revealed a fourth heart sound. The 12-lead ECG showed normal sinus rhythm, left atrial enlargement, and left ventricular hypertrophy (LVH). Chest radiography was unremarkable, and the mediastinum was not widened. Laboratory tests showed elevated highly sensitive cardiac troponin T and serum creatinine levels. A chest CT with intravenous contrast could not be performed due to significantly abnormal kidney dysfunction. What is the most appropriate next step in this patent's management? (See figure in Chapter 10, Case 6.)

Case Review

This case describes the importance of a thorough history and physical examination in the diagnosis of aortic dissection. Uncontrolled hypertension, the pattern of chest pain, unequal pulses, and widened mediastinum are the clinical clues for diagnosis. D-dimer might also be elevated in aortic dissection. The diagnosis can be made by either chest CT angiography, MRI, or transesophageal echocardiography (TEE). In this clinical scenario, abnormal kidney function can be due to either hypertensive crisis or extension of the dissection into the renal artery. The diagnosis can be made by MRI or TEE based on hemodynamic stability. The key is initiation of β-adrenoceptor blockade to control the heart rate and blood pressure as well as to relieve arterial wall stress.

Case Discussion

Aortic dissection is a medical emergency in which a false lumen is created in the aorta due to intimal tear.

Classification

Stanford classification of aortic dissection is as follows: type A involves the ascending aorta and aortic arch, whereas type B involves a tear in the descending aorta, distal to the left subclavian artery.

Risk Factors

- Uncontrolled blood pressure
- Atherosclerosis
- Bicuspid aortic valve
- Aortic aneurysm
- Connective tissue disorders such as Marfan, Ehlers-Danlos, and Loeys-Dietz syndromes
- Inflammatory or infectious conditions such as giant cell arteritis, Behçet disease, and syphilis

Clinical Symptoms

Symptom includes asymmetric blood pressure measurements with unequal pulses, sudden severe tearing chest or upper back (intrascapular) pain, abdominal pain, signs of heart failure such as dyspnea and syncope, peripheral neuropathy, paraplegia, and signs of cardiac tamponade such as pulsus paradoxus.

Diagnosis

Diagnostic evaluation includes chest CT angiography, MRI or magnetic resonance angiography, and transthoracic echocardiography or TEE. Highly sensitive cardiac troponin T, pro-B-type natriuretic peptide, and D-dimer levels are elevated. The 12-lead ECG shows LVH and inferior wall ST-segment elevation myocardial infarction (special circumstances).

Complications

An aortic dissection can lead to:

- Inferior wall myocardial infarction due to extension into the right coronary artery
- Organ damage, such as acute kidney injury or life-threatening intestinal damage
- Stroke
- Acute aortic regurgitation
- Acute heart failure
- Cardiac tamponade

Management

The first-line therapy for patients who are not in obstructive shock includes control of blood pressure. Intravenous β-adrenergic blockers should be used; if additional blood pressure control is required, then intravenous sodium nitroprusside can be added. The heart rate should be targeted to 60 bpm.

   Type A dissection has a very high mortality rate, and emergent surgery is recommended for all patients. Type B dissection is usually treated medically. Surgery is considered for complicated type B dissection (end-organ ischemia), rapid aneurysmal expansion, and rupture or propagation of the dissection. Percutaneous endovascular aortic repair is a convenient, less invasive option for symptomatic type B dissection. Postoperative surveillance imaging is required at 1, 3, 6, and 12 months.

Key Points

- Aortic dissection is a medical emergency that should be considered in the setting of severe chest pain and uncontrolled blood pressure.
- Diagnosis is made by chest CT angiography, MRI, or TEE based on hemodynamic stability.
- Heart rate and blood pressure control is essential using β-adrenergic blockers.
- Emergency surgical repair is required in type A dissection, and medical management can be used in type B dissection.
- Inherited, infectious, or inflammatory causes should be considered in the young population.

CASE 8

Diagnosis of Acute Pericarditis

A 32-year-old man was evaluated in the emergency department for a 5-day history of substernal chest pain. The pain was aggravated by laying in the supine position and improved when leaning forward. Furthermore, the patient mentioned that he had flulike symptoms 10 days ago. He had no other medical or surgical history and takes no medication. On physical examination, vital signs were stable. There were no jugular venous pulsations noted. On cardiac auscultation, the first and second heart sounds were normal. A rub was audible in the left lower parasternal border during end expiration. The remaining physical examination was unremarkable. Laboratory data revealed leukocytosis and elevated C-reactive protein (CRP) and erythrocyte sedimentation rate (ESR) levels. The 12-lead ECG showed diffuse ST-segment elevations with isolated PR interval elevation in lead aVR (as shown in Figure 1.8.1). What is the most important next step in the management of this patient?

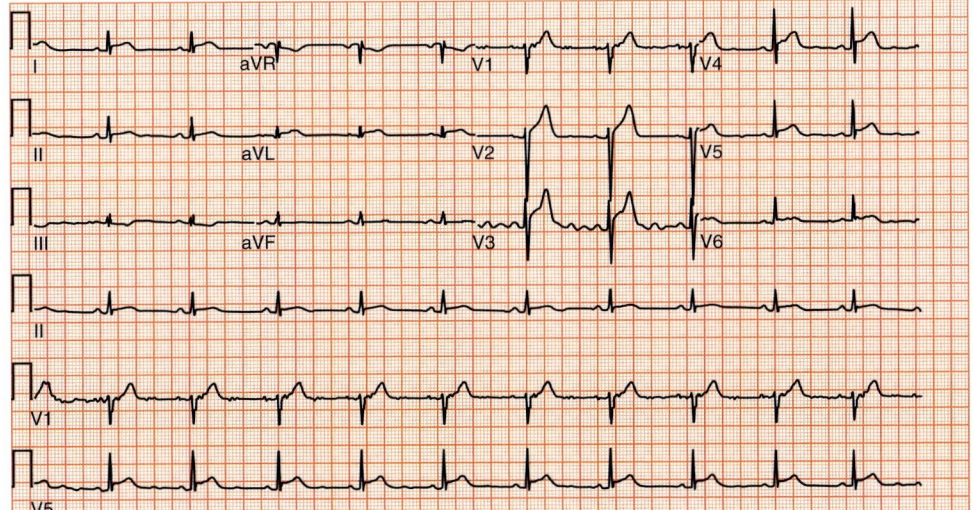

Figure 1.8.1 Diffuse ST elevation in precordial and limb leads with PR depression.

Case Review

In the evaluation of nonanginal pain, acute pericarditis is an important consideration. In this scenario, the age, characteristic symptoms, presence of a pericardial friction rub, elevated serum inflammatory markers, and 12-lead ECG evidence of diffuse ST-segment elevation point to the diagnosis of acute pericarditis. Pericarditis can also occur in the setting of post–acute myocardial infarction and postoperative periods, especially after aortocoronary artery bypass graft surgery.

Case Discussion

Acute pericarditis is an inflammation of the pericardium that can be due to infection, inflammation, or autoimmune etiologies.

Clinical Symptoms

Symptoms include chest pain that is worse with laying supine because the pericardium is stretched; chest pain improves with leaning forward. A pericardial friction rub is the hallmark of acute pericarditis. Three components (triphasic) may be auscultated in atrial systole, ventricular systole, and the filling phase of early ventricular diastole.

Causes

In developed countries, the most common cause is idiopathic. Other causes include autoimmune and connective tissue disorders, viral syndromes, uremia, malignancy, trauma, thoracic radiation, and medications such as hydralazine, isoniazid, and α-methyldopa. In underdeveloped nations, tuberculosis and HIV infections are the most common causes.

Diagnosis

Diagnosis can be made based on the following:

- Pericardial friction rub
- Twelve-lead ECG abnormalities: diffuse concave ST-segment elevations, PR interval elevation in aVR and PR interval depression in all other leads, and electrical alternans
- Elevated CRP and ESR levels
- Transthoracic echocardiography that is usually normal but might reveal a pericardial effusion
- Elevated highly sensitive cardiac troponin T level

Management

Treat the underlying cause, and treat for relief of symptoms. High-dose nonsteroidal anti-inflammatory drugs (NSAIDs) can be used for both analgesia and anti-inflammation (aspirin 650 to 1000 mg every 6 to 8 hours or ibuprofen 400 to 800 mg every 8 hours) with a slow taper over 2 to 4 weeks. Colchicine 0.5 to 1 mg for 3 months can decrease the rate of treatment failure and recurrent pericarditis. Glucocorticoids are reserved for patients who have a contraindication to NSAIDs or those with refractory pericarditis.

Key Points

- Acute pericarditis is diagnosed by clinical history and physical examination findings.
- Elevated inflammatory markers can assist in the diagnosis.
- Characteristic 12-lead ECG changes should be evaluated.
- NSAIDs and colchicine are the treatment options.
- Post–acute myocardial infarction pericarditis should be treated with high-dose aspirin in lieu of NSAIDs.

CASE 9

Management of In-Stent Thrombosis

A 66-year-old man presented to the emergency department with a sudden onset of severe substernal chest pressure associated with diaphoresis and dyspnea for the past 5 hours. The chest discomfort radiated to the left arm and was unrelieved by acetaminophen. He denied any other symptomatology. His medical conditions included coronary artery disease, status post percutaneous coronary intervention (PCI) with drug-eluting stents to the right coronary artery (RCA) placed 2 weeks ago for an acute coronary syndrome (ACS; inferior wall ST-segment elevation myocardial infarction [STEMI]), hypertension, and peripheral vascular disease. He reported compliance with his medication regimen but then stated he missed the past few days because he was busy and forgot to take his medications. There was no significant social or family history noted. In the field, emergency medical services administered aspirin and nitroglycerin, but the chest discomfort was persistent. Upon arrival, the vital signs were blood pressure of 125/80 mm Hg, pulse rate of 45 bpm, respiratory rate of 18 breaths/min, and oxygen saturation of 98% on room air. He was noted to be in acute distress, but the remaining physical examination was unremarkable. The initial 12-lead ECG showed ST-segment depressions in leads II, III, and aVF, with subtle T-wave inversions in V_1 to V_3. He was given morphine, high-dose aspirin, and clopidogrel and begun on an unfractionated heparin infusion. Laboratory data revealed elevated highly sensitive cardiac troponin T with an upward trend. He was taken immediately to the cardiac catheterization laboratory, where he was found to have thrombosis of the RCA stents. He underwent PCI, and revascularization was performed. Subsequently, he was admitted to the telemetry floor. How would you manage this case?

Case Review

In this case, the patient presented with reinfarction likely secondary to subacute stent thrombosis. Noncompliance with medications is a major cause of stent thrombosis. Immediate revascularization should be performed even in cases presenting with ACS (non–ST-segment elevation myocardial infarction [NSTEMI]/unstable angina [UA]) symptoms. Careful identification of the etiology of stent thrombosis should be determined, and conditions such as left ventricular thrombus and hypercoagulable states should be excluded. Another important point is the importance of medication compliance with dual antiplatelet therapy (DAPT) and adequate patient education.

Case Discussion

Stent thrombosis can present as an ACS, cardiogenic shock, or even sudden cardiac death. The cause is multifactorial. Exposure of blood to prothrombotic and subendothelial constituents prior to reendothelialization can trigger the coagulation cascade of events. Furthermore, persistent slow coronary blood flow, inadequate antiplatelet therapy, and the presence of a hypercoagulable state are considered risk factors for stent thrombosis.

A high index of suspicion followed by immediate cardiac catheterization is required in these cases. The 12-lead ECG may show dynamic ischemic changes in the territory of the stented coronary artery but that can extend proximally or distally involving a larger area. It is important to note that not all patients with stent thrombosis present with 12-lead ECG changes.

The Academic Research Consortium (ARC) defines stent thrombosis as follows:

Definite	Angiographic or autopsy confirmation of thrombus in blood vessel
Probable	Unexplained death occurring within 30 days of stent procedure
Possible	Unexplained death occurring after 30 days of stent procedure

Stent thrombosis can be classified based on the time period of presentation since the placement of the stent, as follows:

Classification	Time Period
Acute	Up to 24 hours of stent placement
Subacute	>2 days to 30 days
Late	>30 days to 1 year
Very late	>1 year

Clinical Symptoms

Typical ACS symptoms such as chest discomfort, dyspnea, diaphoresis, dizziness, syncope, and sudden cardiac death.

Management

In patients presenting with an ACS/STEMI, immediate cardiac catheterization and emergent reperfusion therapy are mandatory. However, in patients presenting with an ACS (NSTEMI/UA) in which suspicion for stent thrombosis is high, unlike treating with conservative therapy, urgent coronary angiography and reperfusion therapy should be performed. These patients should be treated with DAPT for at least 1 year. Medications of choice include aspirin plus clopidogrel, prasugrel, or ticagrelor. Patients who develop stent thrombosis on clopidogrel therapy should be changed to prasugrel or ticagrelor. Appropriate follow-up with patient education should be provided.

Key Points

- Stent thrombosis should be suspected when patients present with recurrent ACS after PCI.
- Urgent revascularization is the management of choice followed by long-term DAPT.
- DAPT includes aspirin plus clopidogrel. Any patient who develops stent thrombosis on clopidogrel therapy should be changed to prasugrel or ticagrelor.

CASE 10

Diagnosis of Cardiac Sarcoidosis

A 50-year-old man presented to the emergency department with a complaint of right-sided chest pain for the past week. The pain was described as constant, sharp, 7/10 in intensity, and without radiation, aggravating, or alleviating factors. Other symptoms included dyspnea and wheezing. He has a past medical history of cardiac and pulmonary sarcoidosis diagnosed 5 years ago. In addition, he has a nonischemic cardiomyopathy and underwent placement of an automatic implantable cardioverter-defibrillator (AICD), and he has hypertension and seizure disorder. He is a former smoker but has no other recreational habits. He had been prescribed prednisone by his primary care physician for sarcoidosis but was nonadherent to his medications and follow-up. On arrival, tachycardia was noted. The physical examination revealed diffuse wheezing. The 12-lead ECG showed right bundle branch block (RBBB) without ST-T–wave changes. The patient received aerosolized bronchodilator nebulizers and intravenous corticosteroid therapy with improvement in his symptoms. A chest CT scan with contrast showed bilateral mediastinal lymphadenopathy and diffuse interstitial lung infiltrates. The highly sensitive cardiac troponin T level was normal. The patient was admitted to the telemetry floor for further management. Aerosolized bronchodilator nebulizer treatment was continued and methylprednisolone was begun, and the patient's symptoms improved. How would you manage the case further?

Case Review

An exacerbation of sarcoidosis presents with chest pain or tightness, dyspnea, and wheezing. In this scenario, the patient was diagnosed with an exacerbation based on clinical and physical examination findings along with a normal highly sensitive cardiac troponin T level and lack of ST-T–wave changes on the 12-lead ECG. The characteristic chest CT scan findings are a clue toward the diagnosis. A chronic obstructive pulmonary disease (COPD) exacerbation is a differential in the diagnostic assessment. Furthermore, the patient improved after receiving aerosolized bronchodilator and corticosteroid treatment, which is the cornerstone treatment of COPD.

Case Discussion

Cardiac sarcoidosis is a rare disease in which granulomas are formed inside the myocardium, causing arrhythmias and conduction defects. It can also result in heart failure. Cardiac involvement in sarcoidosis can be difficult to diagnose clinically. Diagnostic testing and its related findings include the following: 12-lead ECG—complete RBBB, arrhythmias, atrioventricular block, and ST-T–wave changes; transthoracic echocardiography—abnormal wall motion and regional wall thinning; thallium-201 myocardial scintigraphy or abnormal accumulation by gallium-67 or technetium-99m—myocardial perfusion defects; cardiac MRI—patchy, multifocal late gadolinium enhancement with sparing of the endocardial border; and endomyocardial biopsy—noncaseating granulomas. Involvement of multiple organs such as pulmonary organs, eye, and integument can also be found, and a multidisciplinary team approach should be adopted for its management.

Clinical Symptoms

Symptoms include chest pain, dyspnea, fatigue, heart failure, palpitation, syncope, and arrhythmias.

Management

The treatment focuses on reducing inflammation and arrhythmia management. Corticosteroids and immunosuppressive therapy such as azathioprine, cyclophosphamide, and methotrexate are used for immunosuppression. Arrhythmias can be controlled with anti-arrhythmic drugs but may require catheter ablation to block abnormal electrical signaling pathways in the heart and AICD implantation.

Key Points

- Cardiac sarcoidosis should be considered if there is significant atrioventricular block, ventricular arrhythmia, and nonischemic cardiomyopathy in patients with no conventional cardiovascular risk factors.
- The diagnosis of cardiac sarcoidosis remains very challenging. Transthoracic echocardiography, cardiac MRI, and positron emission tomography imaging should be performed in patients with a clinical suspicion of cardiac sarcoidosis.
- AICD implantation should be considered early for ventricular arrhythmias due to high risk for sudden cardiac death.
- The extent of left ventricular dysfunction seems to be the most important predictor of prognosis.

2

10 Real Cases on Arrhythmias: Diagnosis of Tachyarrhythmia and Bradyarrhythmia With Management

Nisha Ali • Manoj Bhandari

CASE 1

Management of Second-Degree Atrioventricular Block

A 75-year-old man presented to the emergency department (ED) with the complaint of dizziness for the past week. He denied any chest pain, shortness of breath, tinnitus, hearing loss, or syncope. He has a medical history of hypertension, diabetes mellitus, and glaucoma. His medications included aspirin, pravastatin, amlodipine, hydrochlorothiazide, carvedilol, and timolol eye drops. His dose of carvedilol was increased from 6.25 to 12.5 mg last week by his primary physician. He denied any toxic habits. On physical examination in the ED, he was vitally stable with no significant findings. Initial ECG is shown in Figure 2.1.1. All prior ECGs showed normal sinus rhythm. CT of the head showed no abnormality. The patient was transferred to the telemetry floor where carvedilol was kept on hold. How would you manage this patient?

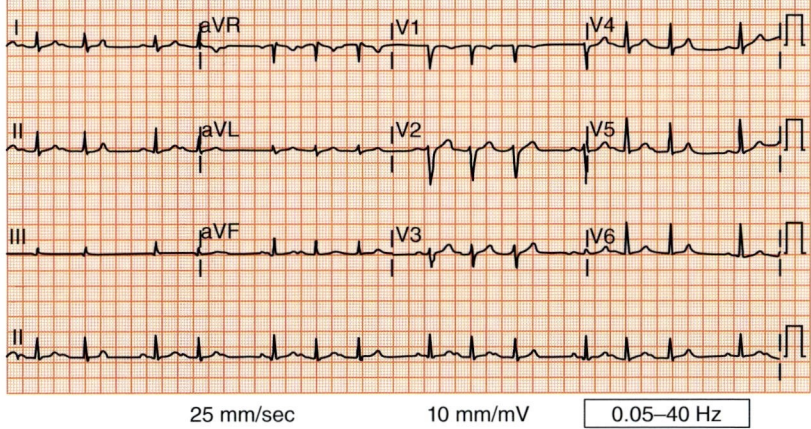

25 mm/sec   10 mm/mV   0.05–40 Hz

Figure 2.1.1 Second degree AV block.

Case Review

This case describes the importance of medication review in the elderly population. Elderly patients taking excessive atrioventricular (AV) node-blocking agents can have symptoms of dizziness and syncope with remarkable ECG changes. The temporal association of the medication dose increase and careful review of the medication list are key to diagnose the etiology of dizziness and AV block. β-Blockers (oral or topical) and calcium channel blockers can be offending agents for this presentation.

Case Discussion

Type II AV block is a disease of the conduction system in which conduction block occurs between the atria and ventricles, leading to 1 or more of the atrial impulses not conducting to the ventricles.

Types of AV block include the following:

- Mobitz type I (Wenckebach phenomenon) second-degree AV block: Progressive PR interval prolongation precedes a nonconducted P wave. The first P wave after block conducts to the ventricle with a shorter PR interval compared with the last P wave before block.
- Mobitz type II second-degree AV block: Intermittently nonconducted P waves not preceded by PR prolongation and not followed by PR shortening.
- High-grade AV block: Two or more consecutive P waves are nonconducted.

Mobitz type I and type II second-degree AV block cannot be differentiated from the ECG when 2:1 AV block is present; 2:1 AV block can be assessed using various maneuverers and pharmacologic testing to categorize the block as Mobitz type I or II. Carotid sinus massage or adenosine slows AV nodal conduction, and with reduction in block from 2:1 to 3:2, Mobitz type I can be revealed. However, atropine and exercise enhance AV nodal conduction and will eliminate Mobitz type I.

Reversible causes include ablation and medications that block AV conduction such as β-blockers, calcium channel blockers, and digoxin. Other causes include myocardial infraction, cardiomyopathy, endocarditis, and myocarditis. A diagnosis is usually made based on history and ECG.

Clinical Symptoms

Symptoms include dizziness, syncope, fatigue, chest pain, shortness of breath, and sudden cardiac arrest.

Management

The management of patients with Mobitz type I second-degree AV block depends on the presence or absence of symptoms. If the patient is asymptomatic, then no intervention is needed. If symptoms are present, then potential reversible causes should be identified such as increased vagal tone, hypothyroidism, hyperkalemia, and medications that block AV conduction. If no cause is identified, then the patient will need a pacemaker. Mobitz type II, however, can progress to complete heart block, and thus a pacemaker is indicated. If the patient is hemodynamically unstable, then the patient should be treated with atropine and temporary cardiac pacing on an urgent basis. In the appropriate clinical scenario, infectious or infiltrative disease may be considered (Lyme disease or sarcoidosis).

Key Points

- Mobitz type I AV block is a disease of the AV node that, in most cases, is secondary to medications and is reversed once medications are discontinued.
- Mobitz type II AV block is the disease of the distal conduction system (His-Purkinje system) and may progress rapidly to complete heart block, leading to sudden cardiac death. The definitive treatment for this form of AV block is an implantable pacemaker.

CASE 2

Management of First-Degree Atrioventricular Block

A 68-year-old man was admitted to the hospital for elective right knee arthroplasty. ECG done postoperatively showed a heart rate of 85 bpm. The ECG is shown in Figure 2.2.1. The intraoperative course was uneventful. He has a medical history of hypertension, hyperlipidemia, coronary artery disease, and right knee osteoarthritis. He denied any chest pain, shortness of breath, dizziness, palpitations, or syncope. He takes aspirin, atorvastatin, metoprolol, losartan, and Tylenol as needed for pain. Based on the ECG findings, the surgeon decided to transfer the patient to the telemetry floor. What further investigation would you do as a result of these ECG findings?

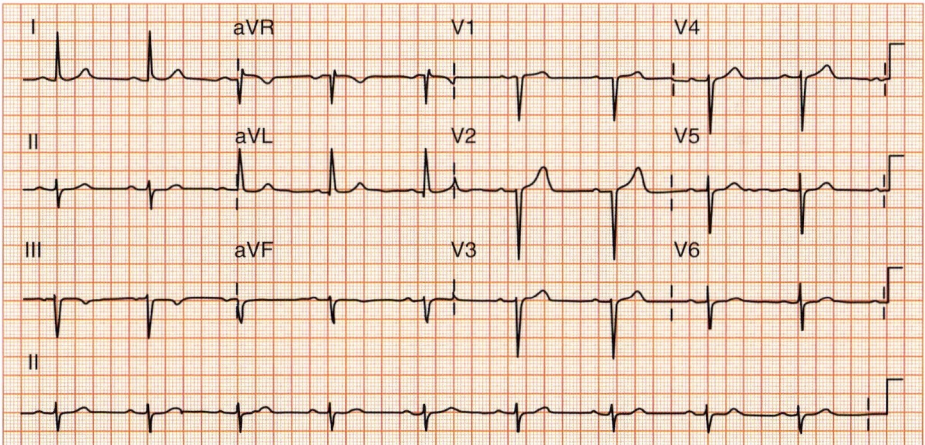

Figure 2.2.1 First degree AV block.

Case Review

This case describes the management of first-degree atrioventricular (AV) block. The ECG findings are incidental, and because the patient is asymptomatic, no further intervention is required. First-degree AV block is a misnomer and is not associated with any pathology. No further treatment is required in this case.

Case Discussion

First-degree AV block is a conduction delay from the atria to the ventricles. It is almost always asymptomatic and is usually diagnosed on ECG (PR interval >200 milliseconds). Physiologically, it could be due to increased vagal tone. Other causes include a structural abnormality of the AV node or medications that slow AV conduction such as β-blockers, digoxin, and calcium channel blocker. It can also be associated with myocardial infarction, Lyme disease, or infiltrative disease (sarcoidosis).

Clinical Symptoms

Patients are usually asymptomatic. If symptoms are present, then signs of bradycardia may be seen.

Management

Asymptomatic patients with first-degree AV block do not require any specific therapy. In rare circumstances, a pacemaker is required when symptoms are consistent with the loss of AV synchrony. In such cases, the indication for a pacemaker device is symptomatic bradycardia instead first-degree AV block. It is also associated with increased risk of atrial fibrillation and increased long-term mortality.

Key Points

- First-degree AV block is benign, often an incidental finding, and rarely symptomatic.
- Asymptomatic patients do not require any therapy.

CASE 3

Management of Ventricular Tachycardia

A 50-year-old man was brought to the emergency department by emergency medical services (EMSs) as an ST-segment elevation myocardial infarction (STEMI) notification. He woke up around 5:00 a.m. with substernal chest pain associated with diaphoresis and dyspnea. EMS was called, and the ECG showed ST elevation in V_1, V_2, V_3, and V_4 (shown in Figure 2.3.1). The patient received aspirin, Plavix (clopidogrel), and sublingual nitroglycerin and was taken to the cardiac catheterization lab where he was found to have a culprit lesion in the left anterior descending artery, for which a drug-eluting stent was placed. He was then transferred to the telemetry floor, where he remained free of chest pain. During the same night, he was noticed to have wide-complex tachycardia on the telemetry monitor that persisted for 30 seconds and then resolved. The patient remained asymptomatic during the event. How will you manage the case?

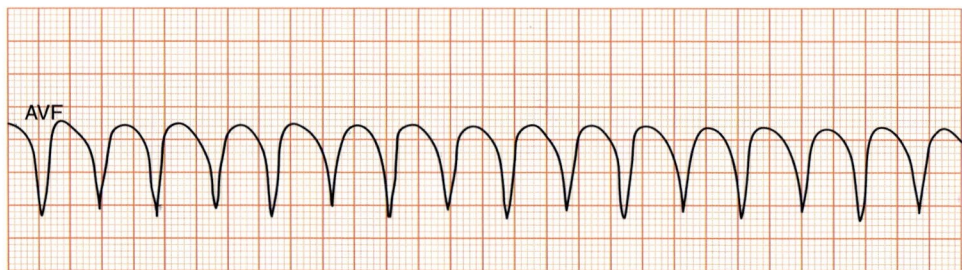

Figure 2.3.1 Ventricular tachycardia.

Case Review

This patient had a STEMI leading to ventricular tachycardia. Ventricular arrhythmias, ranging from isolated ventricular premature beats to ventricular fibrillation, are common in the immediate post–myocardial infarction (MI) period. Ventricular arrhythmias in the setting of acute MI result from injured myocardium (capable of developing reentrant circuits), arrhythmia triggers (spontaneous ventricular premature beats), and modulating factors (electrolytes imbalance).

Case Discussion

Ventricular tachycardia consists of wide-complex tachycardia that lasts >30 seconds. It can be further classified as monomorphic or polymorphic ventricular tachycardia. Most common causes include MI and electrolyte imbalances. Diagnosis is usually made with ECG and telemetry monitoring. Ventricular tachycardia is identified as sustained or nonsustained based on a duration cutoff of 30 seconds.

Clinical Symptoms

Symptoms include sudden cardiac death, palpitations, syncope, dizziness, nausea, and shortness of breath.

Management

Reperfusion arrhythmia within 48 hours of an MI should be observed with conservative management of ischemia and electrolyte abnormalities. Sustained ventricular tachycardia after 48 hours of revascularization should be evaluated for automated implantable cardioverter-defibrillator placement. β-Blocker therapy can be used, and no further treatment is needed if the patient remains asymptomatic.

For ventricular fibrillation and pulseless ventricular tachycardia, immediate cardiopulmonary resuscitation while attaching an automated external defibrillator should be performed. Biphasic defibrillation uses 120 to 200 J of energy, whereas monophasic defibrillators use 360 J.

For monomorphic ventricular tachycardia in unstable patients, synchronized cardioversion with 100 J is performed. For stable patients, procainamide, amiodarone, or sotalol can be used. If drug therapy fails, elective cardioversion is an option.

Polymorphic ventricular tachycardia should be treated like ventricular fibrillation. Polymorphic ventricular tachycardia with a prolonged QT interval can be treated with magnesium, discontinuation of offending medications, and in refractory cases, overdrive pacing.

Electrolyte imbalances should be corrected and monitored closely.

Key Points

- Arrhythmias of ventricular origin are common after reperfusion in STEMI.
- Management of ischemia and electrolytes and observation for 48 hours are required.

CASE 4

Management of Sick Sinus Syndrome

A 70-year-old man presented to the emergency department (ED) with complaint of progressive shortness of breath for the past few months. It was associated with dizziness and fatigue. He denied chest pain, palpitations, cough, fever, or chills. He has a medical history of hypertension, diabetes mellitus, and hyperlipidemia. His home medications included aspirin, pravastatin, sitagliptin, hydrochlorothiazide, and omeprazole. In the ED, the patient was vitally stable, except that his heart rate was 45 bpm. Chest x-ray showed no abnormalities. Laboratory data revealed normal electrolytes, pro-B-type natriuretic peptide, and thyroid panel. His 12-lead ECG showed sinus bradycardia with exit block (shown in Figure 2.4.1). The patient was transferred to the telemetry floor, where it was noted that his heart rate was decreasing to 30 bpm with abrupt increase to 80 bpm and frequent pauses of 3 seconds in between. How would you manage this patient?

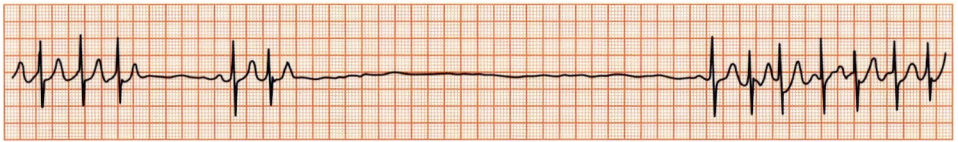

Figure 2.4.1 Telemetry showing heart rate was going down to 30 beats/min with abrupt increase to 80 beats/min and frequent pauses of 3 seconds in between.

Case Review

The clinical presentation and ECG findings are suggestive of sick sinus syndrome (SSS). Most patients with SSS present with nonspecific symptoms such as fatigue, lightheadedness, palpitations, and dyspnea. The medication history, electrolytes, and thyroid studies should be evaluated. Definitive treatment in this case is placement of a permanent pacemaker.

Case Discussion

SSS is characterized by dysfunction of the sinoatrial node. Its etiology includes aging and infiltrative diseases such as sarcoidosis, amyloidosis, and hemochromatosis. Medications such as β-blockers and calcium blockers can also trigger SSS. Other causes include coronary artery disease and hypertension. It is diagnosed by careful history, clinical findings, and ECG. Typical ECG consists of one of the following:

- Sinus bradycardia
- Sinus pauses, arrest, and sinoatrial exit block
- Alternating bradycardia with tachyarrhythmia

If SSS is suspected, Holter or event monitor can be used. Thyroid hormone levels should be checked.

Clinical Symptoms

Symptoms include dizziness, palpitation, chest pain, shortness of breath, fatigue, headache, and nausea.

Management

There are no recommended pharmacologic therapies for patients with symptomatic SSS; however, holding the offending medication can help to avoid symptoms.

Hemodynamically unstable patients should be treated with atropine, dopamine, or epinephrine, as well as temporary cardiac pacing. Stable patients can be monitored with transcutaneous pacing pads in place.

For long-term management, a conservative strategy with watchful observation can be instituted if the patient is asymptomatic. For symptomatic patients, a permanent pacemaker should be placed.

Key Points

- SSS is an abnormal heart rhythm presumably caused by a malfunction of the sinus node and is common in the elderly age group.
- Diagnosis is made by history and ECG and telemetry findings.
- Evaluation for offending causes, such as medications, and thyroid panel should be performed.
- Definitive treatment is placement of a permanent pacemaker.

CASE 5

Management of Asymptomatic Bradycardia

A 41-year-old man presented to the emergency department (ER) with the complaint of fever and cough for the past 2 days. The symptoms were associated with mild shortness of breath and chills. He denied chest pain, dizziness, syncope, or fatigue. His medical history included childhood asthma and gastroesophageal reflux disease, for which he takes albuterol as needed and omeprazole. He lifts weights 3 times a week and jogs 4 miles every other day. His ED vitals revealed a heart rate of 45 bpm, blood pressure of 125/75 mm Hg, respiratory rate of 18 breaths/min, and oxygen saturation of 98% on room air. His physical examination, including a heart and lung examination, was unremarkable. ECG shows sinus bradycardia with no ST-T–wave changes. Chest x-ray in the ED showed right lower lobe infiltrates. He was started on antibiotics and was transferred to the telemetry floor for further management. How would you manage his bradycardia?

Case Review

In this case, the patient was admitted for community-acquired pneumonia, and he was incidentally found to have bradycardia, which is normal in some individuals and requires no treatment. Furthermore, his history of weight lifting and high-endurance training is associated with bradycardia due to increased vagal tone caused by exercise conditioning.

Case Discussion

Sinus bradycardia is described as a heart rate of <60 bpm. It can be physiologic or pathologic. Common causes include advanced age and high-endurance athletic training. Other causes include sick sinus syndrome, pericarditis or myocarditis, head trauma leading to increased intracranial pressure, myocardial infarction, obstructive sleep apnea, atrioventricular (AV) nodal blocking agents (β-blockers, calcium channel blockers), and hypothyroidism. It is diagnosed by an ECG showing a slow heart rate. Furthermore, Holter or event monitor can be used to evaluate the rhythm. Laboratory tests, including thyroid function test and electrolyte abnormalities, can be checked.

Clinical Symptoms

Symptoms include lightheadedness, syncope, fatigue, chest pain, shortness of breath, confusion, and reduced exercise tolerance.

Management

If asymptomatic, sinus bradycardia requires no treatment. If symptomatic, offending medications should be removed, such as AV nodal blocking agents. If it is due to hypothyroidism or obstructive sleep apnea, treatment of the underlying disorder is helpful to improve the bradycardia. Chronotropic response can also be assessed in doubtful cases. For hemodynamically unstable patients, atropine can be administered; if bradycardia does not improve, then temporary cardiac pacing should be considered.

Key Points

- Sinus bradycardia is common in children, the elderly, and athletes.
- For asymptomatic patients with sinus bradycardia, treatment is neither indicated nor required.

CASE 6

Management of Atrial Fibrillation

A 44-year-old woman presented to the emergency department (ED) with a complaint of palpitations for the past 3 hours. She was cooking when she felt that her heart started racing. The symptoms were associated with chest tightness. She tried to take a rest, but the symptoms persisted. She has a history of similar episodes in the past, but they lasted <10 minutes. Her medical history included hypertension and hyperlipidemia. In the ED, the patient was tachycardic with a resting heart rate between 150 and 170 bpm and blood pressure of 140/85 mm Hg. Physical examination revealed irregular pulse and audible heart sounds with no murmur. ECG showed irregular rhythm with no distinct P waves and narrow ventricular complexes (see the figure in Chapter 10, Case 14). Laboratory tests revealed normal thyroid function. The patient initially received adenosine, which slowed down the heart rate, and then 2 intravenous pushes of metoprolol 5 mg, which converted the heart rate to normal sinus rhythm. The patient was then transferred to the telemetry floor. How would you manage this case?

Case Review

In this case, the patient was diagnosed with atrial fibrillation (AF) based on the history, physical examination, and ECG findings. The symptoms of palpitations and typical ECG findings are classic for the diagnosis. In this case, the patient's rhythm converted to normal sinus rhythm after receiving a β-blocker. Furthermore, the patient's CHA_2DS_2-VASc score was 2, and she was initiated on anticoagulation.

Case Discussion

AF is the most common supraventricular tachycardia and is characterized by rapid and irregular beating of the atria. The most common causes include hypertension, coronary artery disease, valvular heart disease, prior heart surgery, congenital heart disease, chronic obstructive pulmonary disease, sleep apnea, obesity, excessive alcohol intake, thyrotoxicosis, and rheumatic heart disease.

Classification

- Paroxysmal AF: AF that terminates spontaneously or with intervention within 7 days of onset
- Persistent AF: AF that fails to self-terminate within 7 days
- Long-standing persistent AF: AF that has lasted for >12 months
- Permanent AF: Ongoing long-term AF

AF can be diagnosed based on clinical history, physical examination (irregular pulse), and ECG (irregularly irregular rhythm with no P waves).

Ancillary testing includes echocardiogram (valves, atrial size, and assessment of left ventricular ejection fraction and pericardium), event or loop recorder (intermittent symptoms not captured on ECG), and laboratory tests such as a thyroid panel.

Clinical Symptoms

Symptoms include palpitations, chest pain or discomfort, shortness of breath, dizziness, syncope, weakness, decreased exercise tolerance, and confusion.

Management

Management of AF includes stroke and clot prevention and rate versus rhythm control. The risk of stroke from nonvalvular AF can be estimated using the CHA_2DS_2-VASc score. The CHA_2DS_2-VASc score consists of congestive heart failure, hypertension, age, diabetes mellitus, stroke, vascular disease, and female sex. Anticoagulation is recommended if the score is ≥2; aspirin is recommended for a score of 1 or when there is a contraindication to anticoagulation. For anticoagulation, warfarin or direct oral anticoagulants (DOACs) can be used in nonvalvular AF. For valvular AF (mitral stenosis and bioprosthetic mitral valve), warfarin is used because DOACs have not been studied in this population.

Rate control is achieved using β-blockers (preferably the cardioselective β-blockers such as metoprolol), nondihydropyridine calcium channel blockers (eg, diltiazem or verapamil), or digoxin.

Rhythm control is achieved using either medications such as amiodarone or electric cardioversion.

In young people with little to no structural heart disease in whom rhythm control is desired, radiofrequency ablation or cryoablation may be attempted.

For hemodynamically unstable patients, synchronized cardioversion should be performed.

Key Points

- AF is the most common supraventricular tachycardia.
- People with AF are more likely to have a stroke than the general population. Clots can also travel to other parts of the body such as the heart, lungs, and kidneys, leading to ischemia.
- If not controlled, over years, AF can lead to tachycardia-induced cardiomyopathy.

CASE 7

Complications in Management of Atrial Flutter

An 82-year-old man was brought to the emergency department (ED) due to a fall. As per the patient, he fell in the morning when he tried to get up after eating his breakfast. He hit his head. He denied chest pain, palpitations, or dizziness. No seizure-like activity was observed. Family members further mentioned that he has become more forgetful over the past few months and has had multiple falls. This is his third fall in a week. Medical history was significant for hypertension, diabetes, and atrial flutter (unsuccessful ablation). Medications included lisinopril, metoprolol, glipizide, and apixaban. In the ED, the patient was found to be confused. Vitals were stable. ECG showed atrial flutter with a heart rate of 90 bpm (shown in Figure 2.7.1). His head CT revealed a 2-cm hemorrhage in the right parietal region. Anticoagulation was kept on hold, and the neurosurgery team was consulted. The patient was transferred to the telemetry floor for further monitoring. On the floor, he had an episode of atrial flutter with rapid ventricular rate, which was controlled by an intravenous push of metoprolol. How would you manage this patient's atrial flutter?

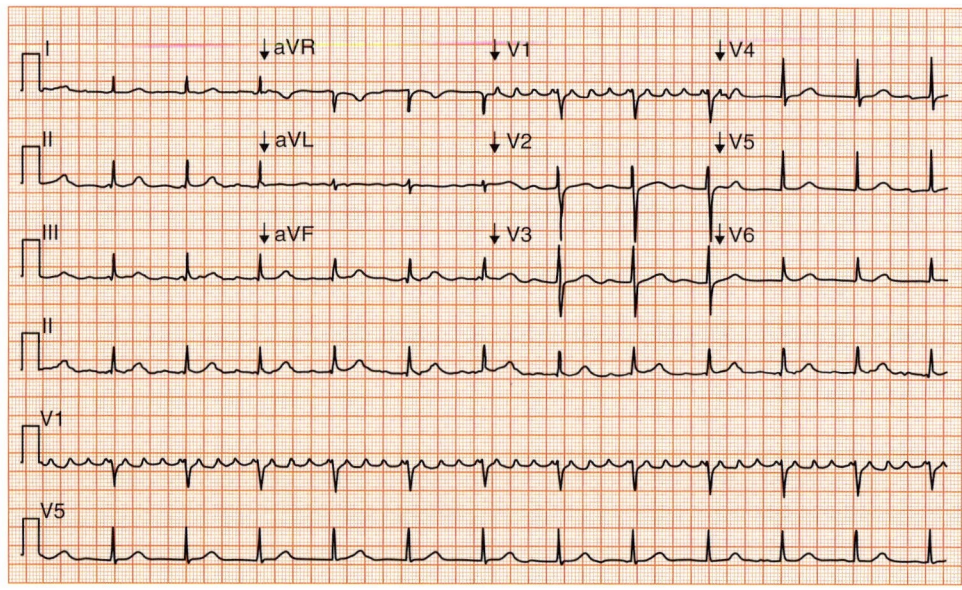

Figure 2.7.1 Atrial flutter with heart rate of 90 beats/min.

Case Review

In this case, the patient has a known history of atrial flutter for which he takes metoprolol and apixaban. Due to the risk of falls in the elderly population, anticoagulation should be used with caution. The HAS-BLED score can be used to assess the risk of bleeding. Goals of care should be decided with the assistance of healthcare proxy. Liberal control of heart rate should be considered.

Case Discussion

Atrial flutter is a form of supraventricular tachycardia with rapid, regular atrial depolarization. Risk factors include coronary artery disease, valvular abnormalities, hypertension, recent cardiac surgery, chronic lung disease, and alcoholism.

Classification

- Typical atrial flutter: Macroreentrant circuit traversing the cavo-tricuspid isthmus (CTI). This isthmus is the region of right atrial tissue between the orifice of the inferior vena cava and the tricuspid valve annulus. The circuit is usually a counterclockwise rotation around the tricuspid valve. If the circuit is clockwise, it is called "reverse" or "clockwise" typical flutter.
- Atypical atrial flutter: This type of flutter can involve any region of the right or left atria other than the isthmus, around areas of scar tissue due to intrinsic heart disease or surgical/ablated scar tissue.

Atrial flutter can be diagnosed with history, physical examination, ECG (atrial rate between 240 and 340 bpm with sawtooth patterns), and echocardiography (evaluate the size of atria and ventricles to look for valvular disease). Further thyroid function testing and an event or Holter monitor can be used.

Clinical Symptoms

Symptoms include palpitations, skip beats, shortness of breath, chest pain, lightheadedness, fatigue, and syncope.

Management

Management of atrial flutter includes rate control and prevention of systemic embolization. Rate control usually involves a β-blocker and nondihydropyridine calcium channel blocker. In some cases, digoxin can be used. Due to the higher chance of recurrence of atrial flutter in patients without a correctable cause, radiofrequency catheter ablation is the definitive treatment.

Patients not responding to catheter ablation or who are not candidates for the procedure can undergo cardioversion using antiarrhythmics, such as ibutilide or amiodarone, or electrical cardioversion. In hemodynamically unstable patients, direct cardioversion should be considered.

Approach to anticoagulation is similar to atrial fibrillation for prevention of systemic embolism. Although the risk of systemic embolism is lower compared to atrial fibrillation, CHA_2DS_2-VASc score should be used to calculate the risk. The HAS-BLED score can be used to assess risk and benefit of anticoagulation. The high-risk factors outlined in the HAS-BLED score are uncontrolled hypertension, abnormal renal and liver function, history of stroke, major bleeding, labile international normalized ratio, age >65 years (elderly), and use of antiplatelet drugs or alcohol dependence.

Key Points

- Atrial flutter can lead to the formation of blood clots in the heart, which pose a significant risk of developing strokes.
- Atrial flutter often degenerates into atrial fibrillation.
- Radiofrequency ablation should be performed because it is mainly resistant to pharmacologic therapy.

CASE 8

Management of Atrioventricular Reciprocating Tachycardia

A 28-year-old woman presented to the emergency department (ED) with complaints of palpitations for the past 4 hours associated with dizziness. She denied any chest pain or shortness of breath. She had been having similar symptoms for the past 2 months, with each episode lasting <10 minutes. She had no significant medical or surgical history. Her family history was not significant for any medical condition. In the ED, her vitals were normal except for her heart rate, which was noted to be 130 bpm. ECG showed delta waves with narrow PR interval. Except for the tachycardia, there were no other significant findings on physical examination. The patient was admitted to the telemetry floor, where the heart rate was noted to be 75 bpm (ECG shown in Figure 2.8.1). How would you manage this patient's tachycardia?

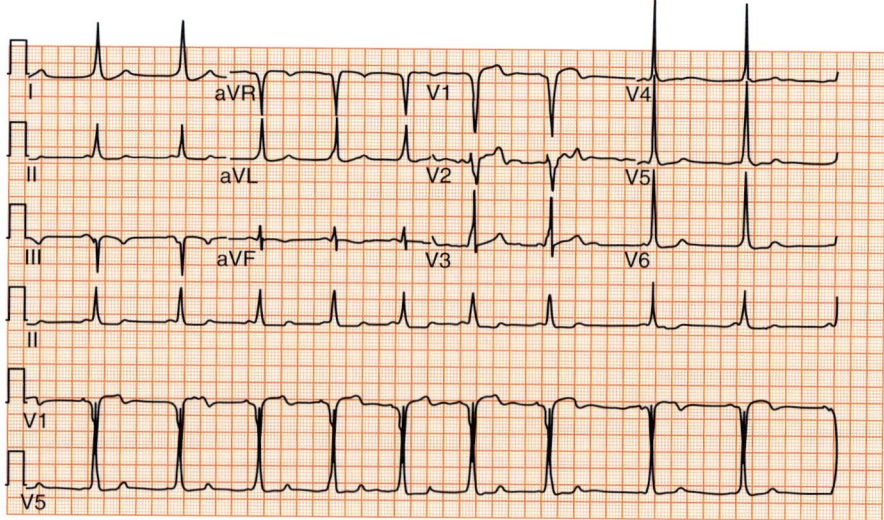

Figure 2.8.1 ECG showed delta waves with narrow PR interval.

Case Discussion

This patient is a young woman with palpitations and delta waves with narrow PR interval, which points to a diagnosis of Wolff-Parkinson-White (WPW) syndrome. WPW is categorized as atrioventricular reciprocating tachycardia (AVRT) with evidence of preexcitation and supraventricular tachycardia (SVT) on ECG. Short PR interval represents electrical conduction via accessary pathways, and delta wave shows ventricular depolarization adjacent to the pathway. AVRT should be evaluated by 12-lead ECG, echocardiogram, ambulatory ECG monitoring, and exercise stress testing. Asymptomatic AVRT (WPW) can be an incidental finding on ECG.

Case Review

AVRT is a disease of the electrical system of the heart in which an extra electrical pathway exists between the atria and ventricles, causing tachycardia.

The cause of WPW is typically unknown. An abnormal gene is the cause in a small percentage of people with WPW. The syndrome also is associated with some forms of congenital heart disease, such as Ebstein anomaly. One-third of cases are associated with atrial fibrillation.

Orthodromic AVRT is the most common type and is associated with narrow QRS complexes and conduction down the AV node. Antidromic AVRT is represented by short PR interval and delta waves. Diagnosis is typically made on ECG or electrophysiologic testing.

Clinical Symptoms

Symptoms include palpitations, dizziness, syncope, shortness of breath, anxiety, fatigue, and sudden cardiac death.

Management

Asymptomatic patients with WPW usually require no treatment. WPW with hemodynamic instability requires synchronized cardioversion.

For orthodromic AVRT, vagal maneuvers such as the Valsalva maneuver, adenosine, or diltiazem can be used. For antidromic AVRT, blockade of the atrioventricular (AV) node is contraindicated, and procainamide, amiodarone, or ibutilide can be used. Use of AV nodal blocking agents in this case can precipitate ventricular fibrillation and sudden cardiac death.

Radiofrequency ablation is the definitive treatment for patients who have symptomatic AVRT, atrial fibrillation with a rapid ventricular rate, or WPW and a family history of sudden cardiac death. In pregnancy, sotalol or flecainide can be used.

Exercise stress testing can be used to assess prognosis in WPW syndrome. Complete resolution of the delta wave is observed in 20% of cases during exercise, which can help to identify patients at low risk for sudden cardiac death.

Key Points

- WPW syndrome is a syndrome of paroxysmal supraventricular tachycardia in patients with short PR interval and delta wave on their ECG.
- The majority of patients with WPW pattern on their ECG remain asymptomatic. It can present as SVT, and AV nodal blocking agents should be used with caution. First-line therapy in stable patients is catheter ablation.

CASE 9

Management of Brugada Syndrome

A 25-year-old man was brought to the emergency department (ED) after he passed out in the college cafeteria for around 5 minutes. He gained consciousness himself, and once emergency medical services reached him, his sugars were normal. There was no seizure-like activity noted. He denied chest pain, palpitations, and dizziness. He had no known medical conditions. There was no history of similar complaints in the past. He reported flulike symptoms for the past day. He denied taking any medications at home. Family history was significant for a father who had a sudden cardiac death at the age of 32. In the ED, the patient was vitally stable. Physical examination was normal. ECG showed elevated ST segment with an upward convexity to an inverted T wave in leads V_1 and V_2 (shown in Figure 2.9.1). Laboratory workup, including troponin and thyroid testing, was normal. The patient was admitted to the telemetry floor for further management. How would you manage this patient?

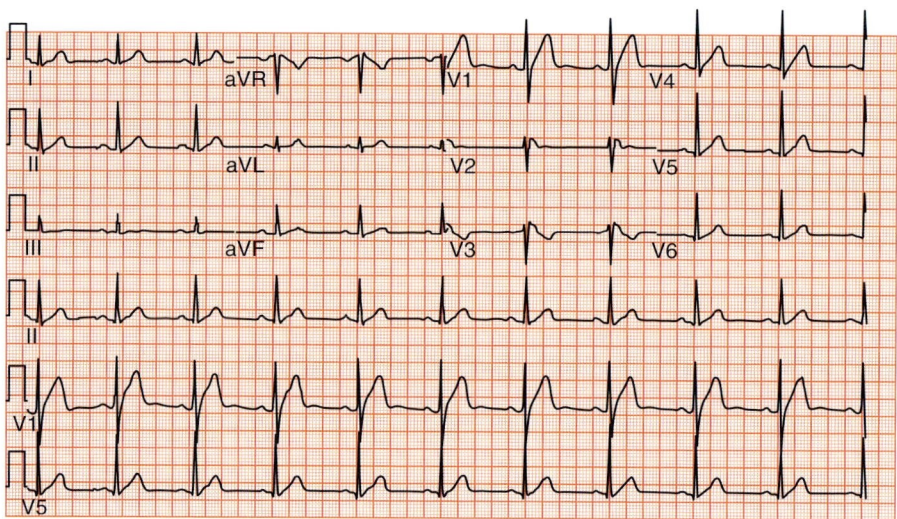

Figure 2.9.1 ECG showing elevated ST segment with an upward convexity to an inverted T wave in leads V_1 and V_2.

Case Review

A young man with a strong family history of sudden cardiac death should be evaluated for inherited arrhythmia syndrome. Sudden collapse in this patient with no anteceded symptoms may indicate ventricular arrhythmia. The characteristic ECG pattern and consistent clinical data point to a diagnosis of Brugada syndrome in this patient, and the patient would benefit from evaluation by an electrophysiologist for automated implantable cardioverter-defibrillator (AICD) placement.

Case Discussion

Brugada syndrome is an inherited, autosomal dominant genetic disorder that can lead to life-threatening ventricular tachyarrhythmias and sudden cardiac death. It is caused by sodium channel mutation. Genetic testing is recommended for all first-degree relatives of patients with Brugada syndrome. It is diagnosed following a clinically significant event (eg, syncope, sudden cardiac death) with typical Brugada pattern ECG findings. However, some asymptomatic patients may be diagnosed based on the presence of ECG findings and relevant family history of sudden cardiac death. The event is typically precipitated by fever or procainamide infusion. Risk stratification can be done by history of syncope. ECG in Brugada can have 2 different patterns:

- Type I: The elevated ST segment (≥2 mm) descends with an upward convexity to an inverted T wave.
- Type II: Saddleback ST-T–wave configuration can be seen, in which the elevated ST segment descends toward the baseline and then rises again to an upright or biphasic T wave.

Clinical Symptoms

Symptoms include dizziness, syncope, sudden cardiac arrest, palpitations, and nocturnal agonal respiration.

Management

An AICD is the mainstay of treatment in Brugada syndrome to prevent ventricular tachyarrhythmias and sudden cardiac death. Patients who are not candidates for AICD can be medically managed with quinidine or amiodarone. Catheter ablation of arrhythmogenic substrate in the right ventricular outflow tract and right ventricular free wall is also an option in some cases.

Asymptomatic patients with Brugada pattern ECG with no family history of sudden cardiac death or a type I ECG pattern do not require any treatment. Brugada pattern with reflex syncope does not require AICD placement.

Certain drugs may precipitate fatal ventricular arrhythmia in Brugada syndrome, and hence, patients and their clinicians should be educated to avoid those medications. Some of the medications to avoid are antiarrhythmic agents (class IA and IC), psychotropic drugs (amitriptyline and desipramine), and recreational drugs (alcohol and cocaine).

Fever is also associated with fatal arrhythmia in Brugada syndrome, and patients should be educated regarding immediate use of antipyretics.

Key Points

- All first-degree relatives of patients with confirmed Brugada syndrome should undergo screening.
- AICD is recommended to prevent life-threatening arrhythmias and sudden cardiac death.

CASE 10

Management of Multifocal Atrial Tachycardia

A 72-year-old woman presented to the emergency department (ED) with complaints of wheezing, chest tightness, and shortness of breath for 2 days. She had a medical history of chronic obstructive pulmonary disease (COPD), hypertension, and diabetes. Her medications included amlodipine, metformin, atorvastatin, albuterol, Symbicort (budesonide and formoterol), and tiotropium. In the ED, her pulse was approximately 130 bpm. Diffuse wheezing was heard on physical examination. ECG revealed irregular rhythm and sinus tachycardia with 3 different morphologies of the P wave (shown in Figure 2.10.1). Chest x-ray showed no infiltrate but hyperinflated lungs. Laboratory workup showed normal troponin and thyroid panel. The patient received dexamethasone and nebulizer treatment and was transferred to the telemetry floor for further management. How would you manage this patient?

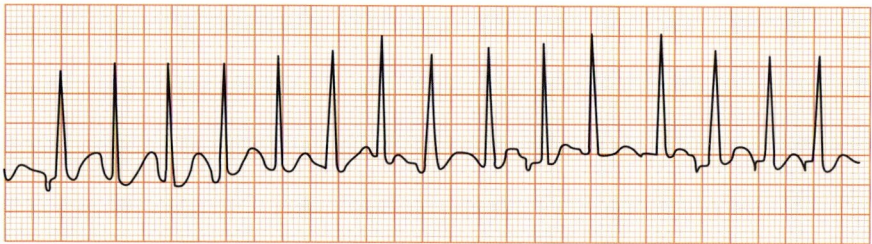

Figure 2.10.1 ECG showing MAT.

Case Review

The case describes a patient with COPD exacerbation who is noted to have tachycardia. The most common causes of tachycardia in these patients are anxiety and albuterol treatment. The presence of different morphologies of the P wave and irregular rhythm should raise suspicion of multifocal atrial tachycardia (MAT). The patient's ECG is suggestive of MAT, which is seen in significant pulmonary disease such as COPD.

Case Discussion

MAT is a rhythm disorder in which the heart rate is >100 bpm with the characteristic ECG feature of variability in ≥3 P-wave morphologies. It is seen in people with significant lung diseases such as COPD, pneumonia, or pulmonary hypertension; coronary/valvular heart disease; hypokalemia; and hypomagnesemia. Diagnosis is usually made based on ECG findings, including P wave with at least 3 different morphologies, heart rate >100 bpm, P wave return to the baseline, and variable P-P intervals, P-R durations, and R-R intervals.

Clinical Symptoms

Patients usually present with symptoms of the underlying disease itself rather than arrhythmias. Some patients might present with palpitations.

Management

Treatment should be aimed at treating the underlying disease. Electrolyte abnormalities such as hypokalemia and hypomagnesemia should be treated. Medical therapy is needed in symptomatic patients with rapid ventricular rate. Medications commonly used are calcium channel blockers and β-blockers (use cautiously in severe bronchospasm). Ablation of the atrioventricular node and the use of a permanent ventricular pacemaker are the treatments of last resort for patients who cannot tolerate pharmacologic therapy.

Key Points

- MAT can be seen in patients with underlying lung disease.
- Treatment should be targeted at treating the underlying condition.

3

10 Real Cases on Syncope and Dizziness: Diagnosis, Management, and Follow-Up

Nikhitha Mantri • Muhammad Saad • Timothy J. Vittorio

CASE 1

Management of Cardiogenic Syncope

A 64-year-old man was brought to the emergency department after an episode of dizziness followed by complete loss of consciousness. According to the patient's daughter, he was resting at home when these symptoms occurred. He regained consciousness within 1 minute without any residual symptoms. There was no history of seizure activity, weakness, or numbness. He denied blurred vision, chest discomfort, and palpitation. His medical comorbidities were uncontrolled hypertension and chronic kidney disease. The medical regimen included metoprolol succinate, lisinopril, spironolactone, and furosemide. There was no significant family history noted. Upon arrival, vital signs were blood pressure of 123/75 mm Hg, heart rate of 37 bpm, respiratory rate of 16 breaths/min, and oxygenation of 95% on room air. The physical examination was notable for sinus bradycardia but otherwise unremarkable. The 12-lead ECG is shown in Figure 3.1.1. The laboratory data revealed potassium of 7.8 mEq/L and creatinine of 2.5 mg/dL. Imaging of the chest and head was negative. How would you manage this case?

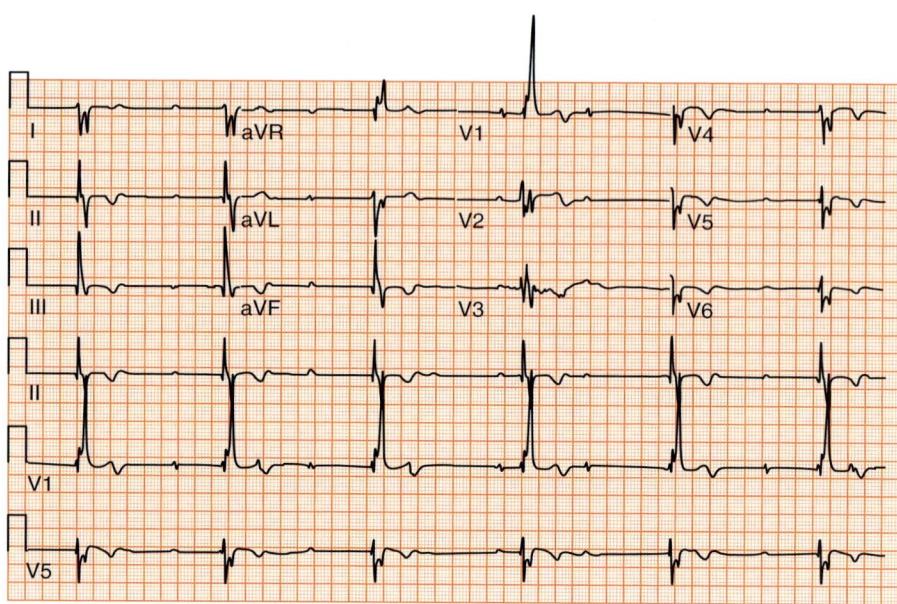

Figure 3.1.1 ECG showing 3rd degree AV block.

Case Review

This patient developed third-degree atrioventricular (AV) block or complete heart block (CHB) secondary to hyperkalemia. The patient has known chronic kidney disease and has been treated with medications including angiotensin-converting enzyme (ACE) inhibitors and mineralocorticoid antagonists, which are known to cause hyperkalemia. Treatment of the underlying cause, particularly hyperkalemia, is important and includes insulin with dextrose, β-adrenergic agonists, such as albuterol, and resin binders. Furthermore, stabilization of the cardiac membrane with intravenous calcium gluconate is a key step in the management of hyperkalemia.

Case Discussion

Third-degree AV block or CHB should be considered as a differential diagnosis in the evaluation of syncope, especially in patients with underlying cardiac diseases. It occurs due to a defect in the AV conduction system that results in the inability of impulses to be conducted from the atria to the ventricles, thereby leading to dissociation of atrial and ventricular contraction. CHB can be due to many conditions, including electrolyte abnormalities such as hyperkalemia; hypoxia; ischemia/infarction; medications such as antiarrhythmic therapy; infiltrative diseases such as sarcoidosis, amyloidosis, multiple myeloma, and hemochromatosis; collagen vascular diseases such as systemic lupus erythematosus, rheumatoid arthritis, systemic sclerosis, and ankylosing spondylosis; infectious diseases such as Lyme disease, Chagas disease, rheumatic fever, and myocarditis; iatrogenic causes such as cardiac surgery; and congenital causes.

Clinical Symptoms

Symptoms of CHB include dizziness, loss of consciousness, chest pain, dyspnea, diaphoresis, and even sudden cardiac death. Occasionally, patients remain asymptomatic or have minimal symptoms. Physical examination findings may include hypotension, bradycardia, and elevated jugular venous pulsations with cannon a waves. These patients commonly present with acute heart failure symptoms.

Management

The 12-lead ECG is characterized by bradycardia and regular P-P and R-R intervals; however, there is dissociation between P waves and QRS complexes. Evaluation of electrolyte abnormalities, toxicology screen, and workup for ischemic, infectious, and autoimmune etiologies should be performed based on suspicion. Transthoracic echocardiography can reveal underlying structural heart disease. Treatment of the underlying cause might reverse the CHB. The management depends on the hemodynamic status of the patient. Advanced cardiac life support measures and temporary pacing (transcutaneous or transvenous) are of utmost importance. Atropine can be also be used as a temporary measure. A permanent cardiac pacemaker should be implanted in stable patients once the offending agent has been discontinued.

Key Points

- Treatment of the underlying cause of CHB and maintenance of hemodynamic stability are important in managing any type of symptomatic heart block.
- Hemodynamically unstable patients with CHB can be treated with atropine.
- Permanent pacemaker implantation is the definitive treatment for refractory CHB.

CASE 2

Management of Dizziness Secondary to Autonomic Dysfunction

A 53-year-old man presented to the emergency department complaining of dizziness for 2 weeks. He reported a "room spinning" sensation, especially when standing up from a seated position. These episodes have been ongoing for the past 2 months but have lately worsened to the point where he is unable to get out of his bed. He denied experiencing nausea, vomiting, blurred vision, loss of consciousness, neurologic deficit, and palpitations. His medical conditions included uncontrolled diabetes mellitus with retinopathy, peripheral neuropathy, and chronic low back pain. There was no significant family or social history noted. Upon arrival, his vital signs showed a blood pressure of 110/90 mm Hg in the supine position and 90/78 mm Hg in the standing position and a pulse rate 82 bpm. The physical examination was unremarkable with the exception of decreased sensation in the bilateral lower extremities (sock-and-glove distribution). The 12-lead ECG demonstrated normal sinus rhythm without ST-T wave changes. Initial laboratory data revealed blood glucose of 240 mg/dL and normal blood cell counts, electrolytes, thyroid function, and liver enzymes. A CT scan of the head was negative. How would you manage this case?

Case Review

This is a case of orthostasis caused by autonomic dysfunction secondary to uncontrolled diabetes mellitus. Assessment of orthostatic vital signs is a key step in the assessment of dizziness and syncope cases. These patients typically present with dizziness on changing positions (postural dizziness). Cardiac and neurologic causes should be excluded based on a detailed history and physical examination. Tight glycemic control is the cornerstone in management.

Case Discussion

Orthostatic hypotension is defined as a decline in systolic blood pressure of 20 mm Hg or diastolic blood pressure of 10 mm Hg or greater within 3 minutes of changing position from the sitting or supine position to standing position. This occurs when the body's normal regulatory mechanisms to maintain blood pressure are unable to compensate with postural changes. There are many causes for autonomic dysfunction, including volume depletion; endocrine disorders such as adrenal insufficiency, hypoglycemia, and uncontrolled diabetes mellitus; neurologic conditions such as Parkinson disease, idiopathic orthostatic hypotension, multisystem atrophy, and Lewy body dementia; and cardiac conditions such as arrhythmias, valvular heart disease, and heart failure. Other causes include drugs, pregnancy, or prolonged immobilization.

Clinical Symptoms

Symptoms of orthostatic hypertension include dizziness, loss of consciousness, generalized weakness, blurred vision, and diaphoresis.

Management

Diagnosis and treatment of the underlying cause are recommended. Assessment of orthostatic vital signs should be performed and is considered high-value care. However, supportive laboratory tests to exclude other etiologies can be considered on a case-to-case basis. Routine testing includes blood cell counts and basic chemistry panel, 12-lead ECG, Holter monitoring, transthoracic echocardiography, and stress and tilt-table testing. Patients with suspicion of neurologic deficit should be evaluated using appropriate imaging studies. The most important part of management is identification of the cause. Hydration, glycemic control, medication reconciliation with avoidance of the offending medication, and use of compression stockings are a few management strategies. Avoidance of abrupt positional changes and use of safety positions should be advised. If conservative management remains unsuccessful, then medications such as midodrine and fludrocortisone can be used with caution. Some of the second-line medications for orthostatic hypotension include nonsteroidal anti-inflammatory drugs, caffeine, and epoetin alfa.

Key Points

- Assessment of orthostatic vital signs is the best and most noninvasive method for the diagnosis.
- Treatment of the underlying cause of orthostatic hypotension is key in management.

CASE 3

Management of Peripheral Vertigo

A 46-year-old man presented to the emergency department with complaints of intermittent dizziness for 2 weeks. He stated that he developed an abrupt onset of dizziness when sitting up and with quick changes in position. The dizziness was described as the "room spinning" around him and was associated with a nauseated feeling and vomiting. He had similar episodes in the past that resolved spontaneously, but this time, the dizziness remained persistent. He denied any hearing loss, tinnitus, focal neurologic deficits, or fever. His medical history was significant for uncontrolled hypertension, for which he takes amlodipine and losartan. There was no significant family history. He denied smoking and recreational drugs but drinks alcohol occasionally. He works as a parking lot attendant. Upon arrival, the vital signs were noted to be stable with negative orthostatic measurements. The physical examination demonstrated vertigo with head movements, especially when sitting up from the examination table and with horizontal nystagmus. The gait was normal. Other cerebellar signs were negative. Head CT scan did not show any acute findings. Initial laboratory data, including blood cell counts and electrolytes, were within normal limits. He was transferred to the telemetry floor for further evaluation. How would you manage this case?

Case Review

This patient presented with intermittent vertigo of 2 weeks in duration. The history and physical examination suggest a positional component with horizontal nystagmus. Presence of intermittent episodes of postural dizziness, nauseated feelings, and negative neurologic signs are suggestive of peripheral vertigo. The management includes head repositioning by various maneuvers and vestibular rehabilitation. Although uncontrolled hypertension can be a cause of central vertigo, other components of the history are not consistent with the diagnosis.

Case Discussion

Peripheral vertigo can be caused by benign paroxysmal positional vertigo (BPPV), vestibular neuronitis, Ménière disease, perilymphatic fistula, vestibular schwannoma, aminoglycoside toxicity, and migraine headache. BPPV is the most common cause and consists of positional dizziness due to an abnormality of the semicircular canals. The onset is usually sudden, lasting for days to weeks, but can sometimes extend for months. The positional vertigo triggers nystagmus when the head is turned to one side. Severity of the disease can vary from mild to severe dizziness even with minimal head movement, and severe disease can be associated with other symptoms such as a nauseated feeling and vomiting. These patients typically have symptom-free periods in between episodes.

Clinical Symptoms

Positional vertigo is the typical presentation in this condition. Nystagmus of limited duration is classic. Severe BPPV will have associated nausea and vomiting. The presence of additional clinical signs and symptoms should lead to further evaluation of other causes of vertigo.

Management

Careful and focused clinical history is the key in the diagnostic approach. Diagnosis is made using the Dix-Hallpike maneuver, which produces nystagmus of limited duration. However, a negative test does not exclude BPPV. The remaining physical examination of these patients is usually normal. The Dix-Hallpike maneuver is performed by changing the patient's head position rapidly from the sitting to the supine positon with head tilted to one side by 45 degrees. The patient is then seated again from the supine position and observed for nystagmus. The procedure is repeated on the opposite side and the patient observed for nystagmus. Other neurologic and otologic causes of vertigo need to be excluded because they can be present concomitantly with BPPV. The treatment of BPPV includes canalith repositioning using Epley maneuver and observation as this condition usually resolves by itself. Other treatment options include medications such as vestibular suppressants, rehabilitation, and surgery. Surgery is usually the last option for refractory symptoms and if the other options remain unsuccessful. Surgical options include labyrinthectomy, posterior canal occlusion, singular neurectomy, and vestibular nerve section.

Key Points

- BPPV typically presents with a sudden onset of positional vertigo associated with nystagmus.
- Vertigo is usually intermittent and precipitated by a specific position.
- Diagnosis can be made using the Dix-Hallpike maneuver.
- Treatment includes the Epley maneuver and observation as this is usually a self-resolving condition.

CASE 4

Management of Syncope Due to Prolonged QT Interval

A 32-year-old man presented to the emergency department with complaints of intermittent palpitation and dizziness for 2 weeks. Additionally, he reported a brief episode of loss of consciousness 1 day ago. He was working but suddenly passed out and regained consciousness very quickly. There were no preceding events, and he never experienced similar symptoms in the past. He denied fever, seizure-like activity, postictal confusion, and any neurologic deficits. His medical history was significant for obesity and sickle cell trait. The medication history included chloroquine, which he recently began taking for antimalarial prophylaxis due to an upcoming trip to West Africa. The family history was negative for cardiac diseases. The social history was negative for any illicit alcohol or illicit drug use and smoking. Upon arrival, the vital signs were within normal range, and orthostatic measurements were also negative. The physical examination was completely unremarkable. The 12-lead ECG showed normal sinus rhythm without ST-T–wave changes and a QTc interval of 536 millisecond. The electrolytes were normal. Toxicology screen was negative. CT scan of the head was normal. The patient was admitted to the telemetry floor. What is the next step in management?

TABLE 3.4.1 Major Drugs Causing Prolonged QT Interval	
Antiarrhythmics	Quinidine, procainamide, disopyramide, flecainide, propafenone, amiodarone, sotalol, dronedarone, dofetilide, ibutilide
Antimalarials	Quinidine, artemether, chloroquine, halofantrine, lumefantrine
Antibacterials	Azithromycin, erythromycin, clarithromycin, roxithromycin, telithromycin, metronidazole, ciprofloxacin, gatifloxacin, levofloxacin, moxifloxacin, ofloxacin, telavancin
Antifungals	Fluconazole, itraconazole, ketoconazole, voriconazole
Antivirals	Efavirenz, lopinavir, ritonavir, saquinavir
Antipsychotics	Chlorpromazine, haloperidol, thioridazine, aripiprazole, asenapine, clozapine, olanzapine, paliperidone, perphenazine, quetiapine, risperidone, ziprasidone
Antidepressants	Tricyclic antidepressants, selective serotonin reuptake inhibitors, trazodone
Miscellaneous	Methadone, buprenorphine, loperamide, ondansetron, domperidone, metoclopramide, donepezil

Case Review

This case projects the importance of drug-induced arrhythmia (acquired prolonged QT interval) in a previous asymptomatic patient. With the exception of obesity, this is a young patient with no other risk factors for cardiac, neurologic, or vasovagal etiologies who presented with intermittent palpitation and syncope of new onset. The recent use of chloroquine, which is known for causing prolongation of the QTc interval, may lead to torsades de pointes and sudden cardiac death. Careful review of the medication history is the key in the diagnosis. Electrolyte assessment, transthoracic echocardiography, and telemetry monitoring should be performed.

Case Discussion

Prolongation of the QT interval is estimated by the 12-lead ECG showing QTc >440 milliseconds in men and >460 milliseconds in women. A patients with a QTc interval >500 milliseconds is at greatest risk for sudden cardiac death. Acquired QT prolongation is separate from the inherited condition and is mainly caused by electrolyte imbalance or medications. Multiple medications are known to cause QT prolongation (Table 3.4.1). Congenital QT prolongation is seen in conditions such as Romano-Ward syndrome and Jervell and Lange-Nielsen syndrome. Other causes such as hypothyroidism, connective tissue disorders, and infections including HIV should be considered. The condition needs to be carefully addressed as it may lead to fatal arrhythmia such as torsades de pointes and sudden cardiac death.

Clinical Symptoms

Symptoms include palpitation, dizziness, loss of consciousness, and sudden cardiac death.

Management

The management mainly depends whether the patient is hemodynamically stable or unstable. The hemodynamically stable patient should be observed on a telemetry unit with serial 12-lead ECG testing after removal of the precipitating agent. Electrolyte imbalances (hypocalcemia, hypokalemia, and hypomagnesemia) should be corrected and drugs prolonging the QT interval discontinued or, if necessary, tapered under a monitored setting. Cardiac monitoring is essential until the QT prolongation is resolved. If the patient develops torsades de pointes but remains hemodynamically stable, intravenous magnesium is the drug of choice. Isoproterenol can be used if the arrhythmia is refractory to magnesium therapy.

In hemodynamically unstable or pulseless patients, the Advanced Cardiac Life Support (ACLS) protocol should be initiated, and unsynchronized cardioversion should be performed. Lidocaine (class Ib antiarrhythmic drug) shortens the QT interval and may be effective, especially for drug-induced torsades de pointes. Class Ia, Ic, and III antiarrhythmic agents should be avoided. Congenital long QT syndrome should be treated over the long term with β-adrenergic antagonists and an automatic implantable cardioverter-defibrillator (AICD) with pacemaker backup. Family members should be evaluated.

Key Points

- Acquired prolonged QT interval should be evaluated with detailed history and medication review.
- Inpatient admission and management with telemonitoring and serial 12-lead ECGs are needed because the patient is at risk for torsades de pointes and even sudden cardiac death.
- Treatment of the underlying cause is of primary importance.

CASE 5

Management of Dizziness Due to Pacemaker Malfunction

A 63-year-old man presented to the emergency department complaining of multiple episodes of palpitation and dizziness for the past 2 to 3 weeks. The dizziness was associated with "spinning of his surroundings" and would occur at any time of the day. He denied a nauseated feeling, vomiting, hearing difficulty, loss of consciousness, and neurologic deficit. His past medical history was significant for hypertension, peripheral artery disease, and prior complete heart block (CHB) status post permanent pacemaker implantation. The medication regimen included losartan, aspirin, atorvastatin, and a multivitamin. The social and family history was noncontributory. Upon arrival, vital signs showed blood pressure of 100/75 mm Hg, pulse rate of 46 bpm, respiratory rate of 16 breaths/min, and oxygen saturation of 98% on room air. The physical examination revealed sinus bradycardia and the presence of a pacemaker generator in the left pectoral fossa, but otherwise was unremarkable. The fingerstick glucose was 110 mg/dL. The 12-lead ECG demonstrated normal sinus rhythm, wide QRS complexes with intermittent pacemaker spikes, and loss of capture. He was transferred to the telemetry floor for further monitoring. How would you approach this case?

Case Review

Dizziness is a common presentation of pacemaker malfunction. There are many causes for dizziness, including cardiac, neurologic (eg, autonomic dysfunction), and iatrogenic causes.

This patient presented with dizziness and palpitations in the setting of bradycardia, and the 12-lead ECG showed improper pacing spikes with lack of capture. This is suggestive of pacemaker malfunction. Pacemaker malfunction should be considered when a cardiac etiology of dizziness/syncope is suspected, and its presentation is quite similar to other cardiac causes. The management depends on correction of the underlying defect associated with the device itself, the leads, or both.

Case Discussion

A cardiac pacemaker is a device that generates electrical impulses to maintain normal cardiac electrical activity. The device includes a pulse generator and leads. Cardiac pacemakers are generally of 2 types: single chamber and dual chamber. Indications include sinus node dysfunction, atrioventricular (AV) block, or other causes of irreversible symptomatic bradycardia. A single-chamber pacemaker (1 single lead placed in either the right atrium or right ventricle) can be used in atrial or ventricular dysfunction, whereas a dual-chamber pacemaker (1 lead in the right atrium and 1 lead in the right ventricle) has a role when AV conduction is impaired but the sinus node still remains intact (See Figures 3.5.1 a-c).

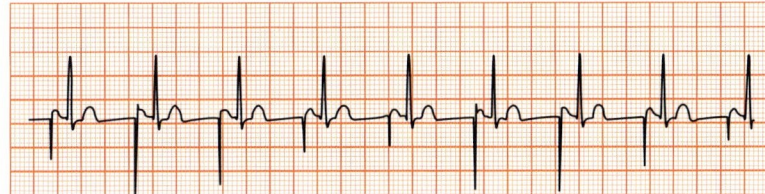

Figure 3.5.1a Single-chamber atrial pacemaker.

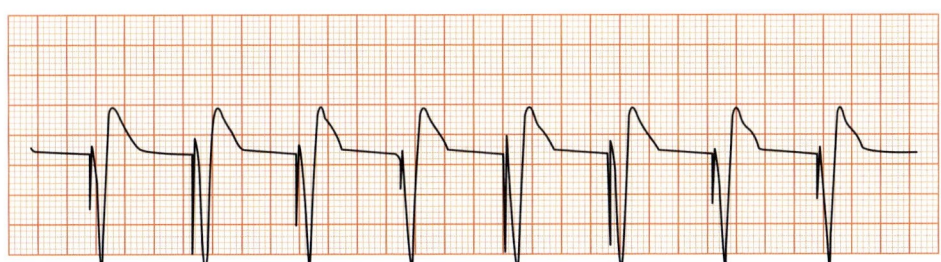

Figure 3.5.1b Single chamber ventricular pacemaker.

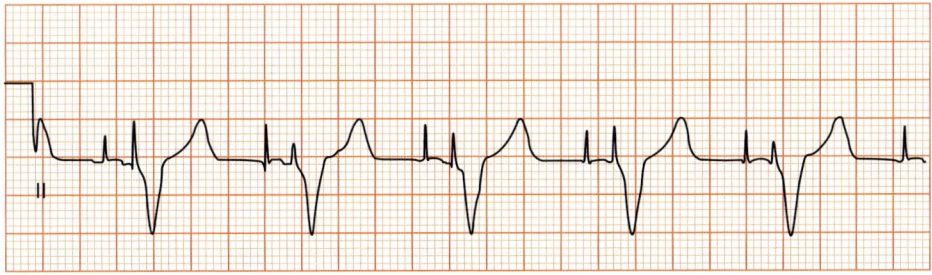

Figure 3.5.1c Dual-chamber atrioventricular sequential pacemaker.

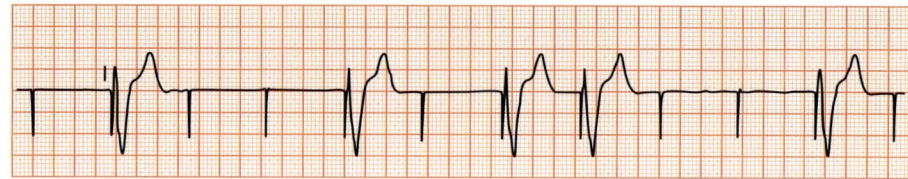

Figure 3.5.1d Over-sensing.

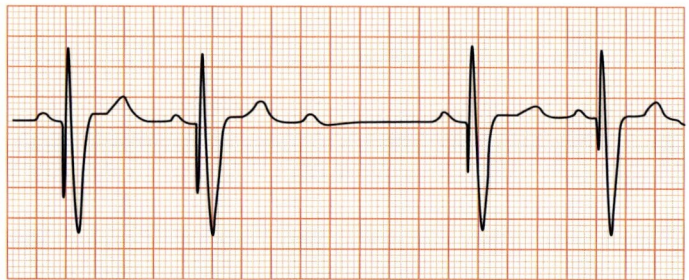

Figure 3.5.1e Under-sensing.

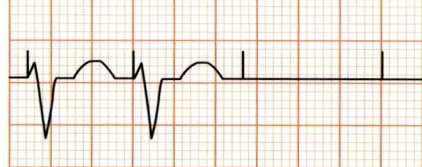

Figure 3.5.1f Failure to capture.

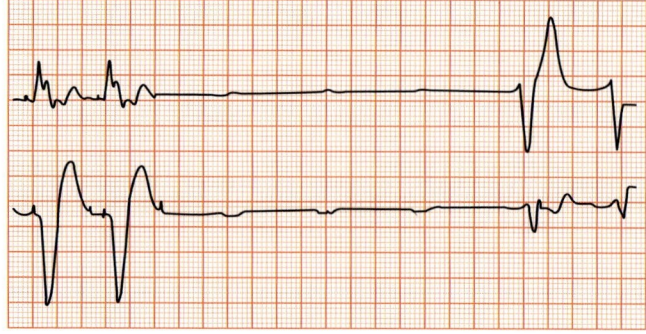

Figure 3.5.1g Output Failure.

A cardiac pacemaker mainly has 2 functions, sensing and pacing. Pacemaker malfunction occurs for various reasons, including malfunction of the pulse generator, leads, or electrode-tissue interface. Most of these malfunctions can be corrected by reprogramming of the device. Occasionally, a device change is required.

Causes of Pacemaker Malfunction

There are numerous causes of malfunction.

- Mechanical causes include generator and battery failure, lead dislodgement, lead fracture, or component malfunction.
- Pacemaker insertion site infection and abscess formation can cause malfunction.
- Other reasons for failure can be due to exposure to high-voltage electricity and high magnetic fields, leading to pulse generator inhibition.

Clinical Symptoms

Symptoms include hypotension, dizziness, syncope, palpitation, and chest discomfort.

Twiddler syndrome is a condition caused by dislodgement of the pacemaker lead and subsequent stimulation of other nerves such as the phrenic nerve, causing abdominal pulsing and hiccups, or the brachial plexus, causing rhythmical arm twitching.

Mechanisms

Mechanisms of malfunction include the following. **Abnormal sensing**, such as oversensing and undersensing, is a common cause of malfunction. Oversensing means that the cardiac pacemaker picks up electrical signals that it should not normally encounter. It leads to the pacemaker sensing it as a normal depolarization rhythm, preventing the cardiac pacemaker from firing a pacing stimulus. Fewer than normal pacemaker spikes are seen on the 12-lead ECG (Figure 3.5.1d). Undersensing occurs when the cardiac pacemaker fails to sense the normal depolarization rhythm and initiates a pacemaker rhythm causing asynchronous pacing. This is seen on the 12-lead ECG as numerous pacemaker spikes (Figure 3.5.1e).

Failure in pacing the cardiac chamber can occur either due to capture failure or output failure. Failure to capture means that the pacing event failed to generate a cardiac impulse. This is seen on the 12-lead ECG by pacemaker spikes but the absence of a depolarization wave of the pacing chamber (Figure 3.5.1f). Output failure occurs when no cardiac pacemaker stimulus occurs even when the heart beats at a lower rate than the set rate. No pacemaker spikes are seen on the 12-lead ECG (Figure 3.5.1g).

Other mechanisms include inappropriate rapid pacing rates, such as a runway pacemaker, which can lead to hemodynamic instability.

Management

There is limited role for medical therapy for this condition. Symptomatic patients with hemodynamic instability should be treated with fluids and transcutaneous pacing. Surgical exploration of the pacemaker pocket; replacement or repair of leads, battery, pulse generators, or connectors; and removal of air from dry pockets are usually recommended. Repositioning of the lead or pulse generator is required in Twiddler syndrome.

Key Points

- Pacemaker malfunction should be considered as one of the causes of dizziness and can present with symptoms similar as any other cardiac conditions.
- Management includes maintaining hemodynamic stability and correcting the underlying defect causing the malfunction.

CASE 6

Management of Hypertrophic Cardiomyopathy

A 24-year-old woman without any medical comorbidities was brought to the emergency department with a complaint of collapsing during a morning jog. After a few minutes, she regained consciousness. She denied chest pain, blurred vision, or confusion, and there were no witnessed seizures. However, there is a history of intermittent palpitation with exertion. The family history was notable for sudden cardiac death (SCD) in her father at the age of 36 years. She denied any toxic habits. She was not taking prescription or over-the-counter medications. Upon arrival, the vital signs showed a blood pressure of 110/75 mm Hg, pulse rate of 75 bpm, and respiratory rate of 16 breaths/min. The physical examination was completely unremarkable. The 12-lead ECG revealed normal sinus rhythm with left ventricular hypertrophy (LVH), as shown in Figure 3.6.1. Initial laboratory testing including electrolytes, blood cell counts, and thyroid panel was normal. High-sensitivity cardiac troponin T was slightly elevated with a downward trend. Drug toxicology screening was negative. CT scan of the head was unremarkable. The patient was admitted to the telemetry floor. The 12-lead ECG revealed normal sinus rhythm with left ventricular hypertrophy (LVH), as shown in Figure 3.6.1. How would you manage this case?

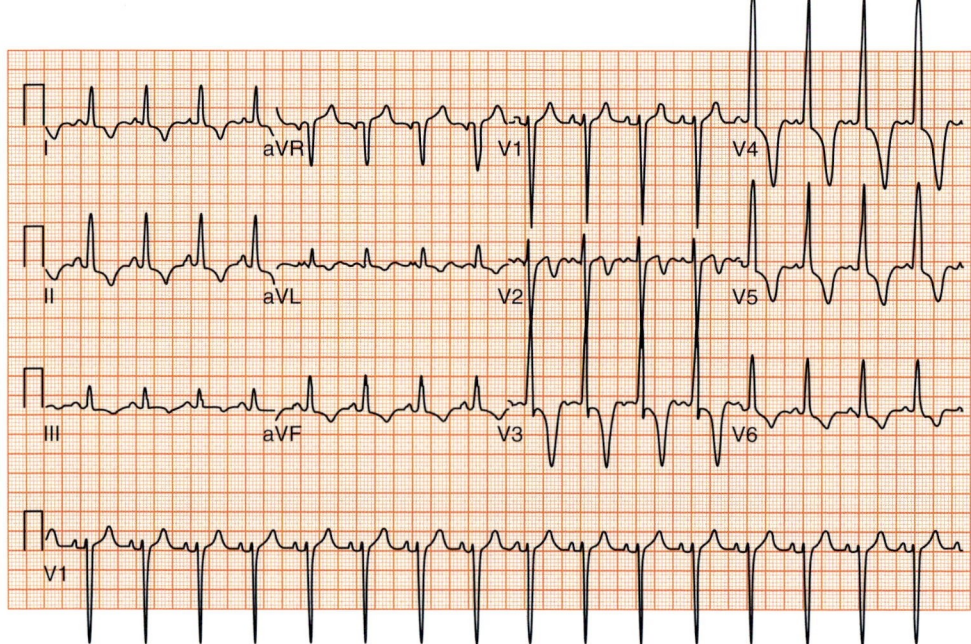

Figure 3.6.1 The 12-lead ECG revealed normal sinus rhythm with LVH.

Case Review

Hypertrophic cardiomyopathy (HCM) should be considered when a young, otherwise healthy patient presents with syncope of unknown etiology. Careful history and physical examination should be performed because this condition can be associated with SCD or have long-term consequences such as heart failure. The family history is an important component of the diagnostic process. An automated implantable cardioverter-defibrillator (AICD) should be placed to prevent ventricular arrhythmias related to SCD.

Case Discussion

HCM is characterized by LVH of unknown cause. The disease has an autosomal dominant inheritance pattern with sporadic cases in rare circumstances. Multiple sarcomere mutations have been identified. The prognosis of HCM is highly variable, from normal life expectancy without disability to SCD. Thus, it is advisable to screen all first-degree relatives of patients with HCM to avoid the risk of SCD in this population. The underlying pathology mainly includes left ventricular outflow tract (LVOT) obstruction due to systolic anterior motion (SAM) of the mitral valve and diastolic dysfunction caused by the hypertrophied left ventricular walls. The LVH can lead to myocardial ischemia due to demand-supply mismatch and arrhythmias.

HCM should be differentiated from other cardiac conditions associated with LVH, including aortic stenosis, hypertensive heart disease, athlete's heart, storage disorders, and infiltrative heart disease. A detailed history and physical examination can help distinguish these disorders.

- Aortic stenosis (AS) usually occurs in the older population. On cardiac auscultation, a classic crescendo-decrescendo systolic murmur with radiation toward the neck and precordium is auscultated. Transthoracic echocardiogram is one of the best diagnostic tests for AS.
- Hypertensive heart disease is a condition where long-standing uncontrolled hypertension leads to LVH and ventricular stiffness.
- Athlete's heart is a nonpathologic condition seen commonly in sports medicine. It is seen in athletes and is a physiologic hypertrophy caused by repetitive cardiac loading. It is one of the conditions that is most often confused with HCM. It can be differentiated from HCM based on absence of family history, absence of genetic mutations, diastolic function, and the LVH pattern.

Clinical Symptoms

The clinical presentation of HCM varies from completely asymptomatic to SCD. Symptoms include dizziness, syncope, exertional dyspnea, palpitation, angina, arrhythmias, heart failure, and SCD.

Management

Cardiac imaging using standard transthoracic echocardiogram is the typical tool used for diagnosis. Cardiac MRI (cMRI) can be used in case of uncertainty. Genetic testing is used for definitive diagnosis of HCM. A 12-lead ECG is usually recommended during the initial evaluation. Holter monitoring or event recording is recommended for patients who present with palpitation or dizziness to detect underlying arrhythmias.

Patients should undergo risk stratification for SCD. Major risk factors include non-sustained spontaneous ventricular tachycardia (VT), blunted blood pressure response to exercise, unexplained syncope, SCD (ventricular fibrillation), family history of premature SCD, and heart failure that has progressed to dilated cardiomyopathy with ejection fraction ≤35% and New York Heart Association class II or III symptoms. These patients will benefit from AICD therapy.

Management of HCM includes genetic counseling and pharmacologic and surgical therapies. For patients who have symptoms such as angina or dyspnea, β-adrenergic antagonists are the drug of choice. Nondihydropyridine calcium antagonists can be used in patients who are intolerant to β-adrenergic antagonists or if β-adrenergic antagonists are contraindicated. Disopyramide can be used carefully in cases refractory to β-adrenergic and nondihydropyridine calcium antagonists. It is recommended to avoid positive inotropic drugs and high-dose diuretic therapy because symptoms may worsen. Patients who present with symptomatic heart failure and reduced ejection fraction should be treated with β-adrenergic antagonists, angiotensin-converting enzyme inhibitors or angiotensin receptor blockers, mineralocorticoid antagonists, and diuretics. Patients who develop sustained VT with prior SCD benefit from AICD placement.

Septal ablation or septal reduction therapy and surgical myectomy are recommended for patients who do not respond to or are refractory to medical therapy. Generally, alcohol septal ablation therapy is preferred as it is less invasive and promotes earlier recovery. Septal ablation is recommended in older adults, especially when surgical myectomy is contraindicated. Surgical myectomy is preferred in younger adults. Orthotopic heart transplantation can be considered in HCM patients with advanced heart failure symptoms who are refractory to all available HCM treatments and with left ventricular ejection fractions ≤50%.

Screening is indicated in all first-degree family members of patients with HCM. The 12-lead ECG, transthoracic echocardiogram, and cMRI can be used as screening tools. Screening generally starts at the age of 12 years, with a frequency of every 12 to 18 months. After age 18 to 21 years, screening is recommended once every 5 years.

Key Points

- HCM should be considered as a differential diagnosis when young, otherwise healthy patients present with syncope of unknown etiology.
- Clinical history and physical examination typically exclude other diagnoses. The key differential diagnoses include hypertensive heart disease and athlete's heart.
- Alcohol septal ablation and AICD implantation are the cornerstones in management.
- Family members should be screened by 12-lead ECG and transthoracic echocardiography.

CASE 7

Management of Pseudosyncope and Migraine-Related Syncope

A 22-year-old woman was brought to the emergency department complaining of sudden loss of consciousness when she was at home. After 5 minutes, she regained consciousness. Prior to the syncopal episode, she complained of severe cephalgia associated with a nauseated feeling and dizziness. Additionally, she described a blackout phenomenon as well as a strange sensation in the abdomen. She reported having recurrent cephalgia for >1 year, sometimes lasting a few hours to 2 days. She administered herself ibuprofen, but it did not alleviate her symptoms. She denied any stress, fever, neurologic deficit, palpitations, and photophobia. Her appetite has been adequate. The past medical history included migraine headache and iron deficiency anemia. The family and social histories were noncontributory. Upon arrival, the vital signs, including orthostatic measurements, were normal. The fingerstick blood glucose was 90 mg/dL. The rest of the physical examination was normal, including the cardiac, neurologic, and ophthalmologic examinations. Initial laboratory data including electrolytes, renal function, and thyroid studies were normal. The 12-lead ECG revealed normal sinus rhythm with no ischemic changes. Urine pregnancy test, drug toxicology screen, and CT scan of the head were unremarkable. The patient was admitted to the telemetry floor. How would you approach this case?

Case Review

Nearly one-third of patients with migraine headache present with syncope. This case described a young patient who presented with syncope, intermittent cephalgia, and aura symptoms, which is typical for migraine headache. The other differential diagnoses in this case are subarachnoid hemorrhage, meningitis, and multiple sclerosis, which should be excluded clinically. Another important differential diagnosis in this case is pseudosyncope, which is precipitated by stress and should be excluded.

Case Discussion

Pseudosyncope is a psychogenic condition often found in young woman that is associated with recurrent loss of consciousness with longer duration and closed eyes. The diagnosis is usually made by exclusion and by recording the event during a tilt-table test with simultaneous blood pressure, heart rate monitoring, and video electroencephalography.

Complex migraine, an overlapping differential with pseudosyncope, can present with symptoms such as neurologic deficits, syncope, cervical pain, and Horner syndrome. The pathophysiology behind migraine headache is unknown but is thought to have a strong genetic component. The key features include recurrent cephalgia associated with aura that includes sensory, visual, tactile, or auditory symptoms. It is more common in women. The headache is typically described as throbbing, unilateral or bilateral, and lasting for few days. It is triggered by known factors such as medication (oral contraceptives), menstruation, smoking, poor sleep hygiene, specific odors, hunger, exposure to excessive/bright light, and certain foods, including caffeine, wine, chocolate, and tyramine-containing products.

Clinical Symptoms

Patients present with typical or atypical headache. Other associated symptomatology includes nauseated feeling, vomiting, dizziness, syncope, and sensory, motor, and visual deficits based on the severity and complexity.

Management

The diagnosis is based on history. No further testing is required unless other conditions are suspected. The management includes both nonpharmacologic and pharmacologic treatments. Nonpharmacologic treatment includes cognitive-behavioral therapy, biofeedback, and relaxation techniques, which are effective in many cases. Pharmacologic treatment of complex migraine includes prophylactic and abortive therapies. Abortive therapy includes nonsteroidal anti-inflammatory drugs, triptans, and opiates based on the severity. Prophylactic therapy includes β-adrenergic antagonists, nondihydropyridine calcium antagonists (verapamil), tricyclic antidepressants, valproic acid, and topiramate. Psychogenic pseudosyncope can be treated with psychotropic medications. The prophylactic medication can be chosen based on the patient's tolerance and presence of concurrent comorbidities.

Key Points

- Pseudosyncope and complex migraine are the rare differential diagnoses in the evaluation of syncope and remain the diagnoses of exclusion.
- Tilt-table testing, electroencephalography, and transcranial Doppler imaging can be performed based on suspicion.
- Cognitive-behavioral therapy and treatment of migraine headache are key elements in the management.

CASE 8

Management of Disequilibrium

An 85-year-old woman residing in a skilled nursing facility was brought to the emergency department with complaints of dizziness and generalized weakness for the past several months. The symptoms have progressively worsened, and she now has a fear of walking. Approximately 3 months ago, she had a prolonged hospitalization for distributive shock secondary to urosepsis. During that admission, she was evaluated by physical therapy on a daily basis and was provided a cane for assistance upon discharge. She denied fever, nausea, vomiting, neurologic deficit, and recent falls. Her other medical conditions included hypertension, dyslipidemia, chronic kidney disease, and osteoarthritis. The family and social histories were unremarkable. The active medical regimen included acetaminophen, nifedipine extended release, aspirin, and pravastatin. Upon arrival, the vital signs were noted as blood pressure of 140/80 mm Hg, pulse rate of 80 bpm, respiratory rate of 16 breaths/min, and oxygen saturation of 98% on room air; in addition, the patient was afebrile. Orthostatic measurements were negative. The physical examination showed a thin elderly woman. The neurologic assessment demonstrated 4/5 muscle weakness in the lower extremities. Additionally, she was noted to have hearing difficulty, visual acuity was 20/200, and the gait was unsteady using a cane for assistance. Initial laboratory data including blood cell count, electrolytes, vitamin B_{12} level, and thyroid panel were normal. The 12-lead ECG revealed normal sinus rhythm with left ventricular hypertrophy (LVH). The patient was admitted to the telemetry floor for further evaluation. How would you approach this case?

Case Review

This case describes the management of disequilibrium as a cause of dizziness in the elderly. This elderly woman with a relatively recent prolonged hospitalization and hearing and vision impairment may be deconditioned, which is contributing to the dizziness. The medication regimen should be carefully reviewed for any over-the-counter medications. Hearing and visual assistance should be provided. Physical therapy has a key role in rehabilitation and gait training. Further cardiac and neurologic testing is unnecessary given the clinical history and physical examination findings.

Case Discussion

Disequilibrium is an underrecognized clinical condition that is especially observed in the elderly population and is associated with an unsteady gait, fear of falling, and inability to ambulate. The common causes include hearing or visual impairment, musculoskeletal disease such as osteoarthritis, lack of proprioception such as diabetic neuropathy, prolonged bedridden state, polypharmacy (use of β-adrenergic antagonist eye drops or diuretics), illicit drug use, cerebellar disorders, and psychiatric diseases. There can be other environment-related causes such as uneven surfaces, stairs, and darkness.

Clinical Symptoms

Symptoms include dizziness/lightheadedness, unsteady gait, difficulty standing, and fatigue with walking.

Management

Disequilibrium can be diagnosed by a detailed history and physical examination. Careful review of the active medication list and medical comorbidities, orthostatic vital sign measurements, and home safety assessment should be performed. Otoneurologic and visual testing should be performed. The Timed Up and Go test can be performed as a bedside assessment in which the patient is asked to stand up, walk 3 m, walk back, and sit back down, which should not take >20 seconds. Physical therapy is used to strengthen the muscles and is an essential component of gait training and selection of medical equipment for ambulation. Posturography testing is an instrument used by physical therapists to evaluate balance disturbances in standing, walking, swaying, and climbing surfaces. Neurologic and cardiovascular testing is often not needed and should be excluded by clinical correlation. Dietary evaluation for calcium and vitamin D should be considered. Appropriate shoe size, use of 2 different spectacles for presbyopia, and use of hearing aids for presbycusis assist in reducing falls. An assessment of the home environment should be performed by an expert physiatrist with appropriate changes made to prevent falls.

Key Points

- Disequilibrium is a clinical condition found in the elderly population associated with an unsteady gait and dizziness.
- Careful review of the medication list and comorbid conditions should be performed and addressed as necessary.
- Physical therapy should be used to strengthen the muscles of ambulation and to prevent falls.

CASE 9

Diagnosis of Alcohol Withdrawal Syndrome

A 45-year-old man was brought to the emergency department by the police after being found wandering the streets with bizarre behavior. The past medical history was unknown. Upon arrival, he was found confused and disoriented with anxiety and tremulousness. The vital signs were notable for blood pressure of 140/95 mm Hg, heart rate of 110 bpm, temperature of 98°F, and oxygen saturation of 98% on room air. Suddenly, he developed a generalized tonic-clonic seizure for which intravenous lorazepam was administered. The cardiovascular, respiratory, and further neurologic examinations did not show any significant findings. His routine laboratory tests showed normal complete blood count. The basic metabolic panel showed low serum potassium and magnesium with normal creatinine. The alcohol level was significantly elevated. The urine and serum drug screening were negative. A head CT scan was normal. Subsequently, he was admitted to the telemetry floor for further management. How would you manage this case?

Case Review

This scenario highlights the management of alcohol withdrawal syndrome. The presence of symptoms such as agitation and anxiety along with hypertension and tachycardia point toward substance use. The onset of seizure activity is also the sequela of symptoms. Although other causes should be considered, including metabolic and septic encephalopathy, the clinical history is essential to exclude the differential diagnosis.

Case Discussion

Alcohol withdrawal syndrome consists of a constellation of symptoms that occurs within 6 to 48 hours of alcohol cessation, usually seen in the setting of chronic alcohol use. Alcohol acts on the γ-aminobutyric acid (GABA) receptors and causes central nervous system depression. Delirium tremens (DTs) occurs 48 to 96 hours after the last drink and can persist for months.

Clinical Symptoms

The symptoms consist of agitation, anxiety, confusion, tremulousness, hypertension, tachycardia, seizures, hallucination, nausea, vomiting, and insomnia. DTs occurs in the setting of fever, hypertension, hallucination, and seizure activity.

Management

The management of alcohol withdrawal syndrome consists of supportive therapy, detoxification, and avoidance of DTs. Therapy is guided by the Clinical Institutes Withdrawal Assessment for Alcohol Withdrawal (CIWA-Ar) tool, with a low score (0 to 9) indicating minimal withdrawal, a moderate score (10 to 19) indicating moderate withdrawal, and a score >20 indicating impending DTs. Supportive measures include quiet environment, intravenous hydration with dextrose-rich fluids, thiamine, folic acid, and multivitamins. Benzodiazepines (BZPs) play a pivotal role in treating withdrawal and avoiding DTs. Short-acting and long-acting BZPs can be used as guided by the CIWA-Ar score, and symptom-based therapy (SBT) should be preferred. Lorazepam, oxazepam, and midazolam are short-acting BZPs, and chlordiazepoxide and diazepam are long-acting BZPs. In severe liver disease, long-acting BZPs should be avoided. Mild symptoms can be treated on an outpatient basis. Nutrition should be initiated early, and oversedation should be avoided. DTs can be initially treated with BZPs, but if needed, haloperidol, propofol, and phenobarbital can be used with monitoring of the respiratory status. Alcohol-related seizures should also be treated with BZPs. Other antiseizure medications are generally not required. Electrolyte monitoring and replacement should be considered, and caution should be raised for refeeding syndrome.

Components of the CIWA-Ar score include the following:

- Nausea and vomiting grading—7 points
- Tremor grading—7 points
- Paroxysmal sweating—7 points
- Tactile disturbance—7 points
- Auditory disturbance—7 points
- Visual disturbance—7 points
- Anxiety grading—7 points
- Agitation—7 points
- Orientation/clouding of sensorium—7 points

Key Points

- Alcohol withdrawal syndrome is a clinical syndrome that occurs 6 to 48 hours after alcohol use.
- Anxiety, confusion, and tremors are major symptoms.
- Supportive therapy includes intravenous hydration and thiamine administration.
- BZPs are the main treatment of choice.
- Electrolytes and nutrition should be adequately replenished.

CASE 10

Management of Neurogenic Syncope

A 27-year-old woman was brought to the emergency department after an episode of witnessed seizure activity 4 hours ago while she was watching television. As per her husband, she started feeling nauseated and suddenly developed a jerking movement of the whole body for a few seconds. Subsequently, she lost consciousness. Her husband called 911 immediately, but by the time emergency medical services arrived, she had regained consciousness but was in a confused state. She denied fever, cough, cephalgia, prior seizure events, weakness, and numbness. Her medical conditions included iron deficiency anemia. The family history was significant for a younger brother with a seizure disorder since the age of 16 years. There was no history of alcohol or illicit drug use. She works as an office secretary. In the field, the fingerstick blood glucose was noted to be 95 mg/dL. Upon arrival, vital signs were blood pressure of 110/75 mm Hg, pulse rate of 85 bpm, and respiratory rate of 16 breaths/min, and the patient was afebrile. The physical examination, including cardiovascular and neurologic assessments, was completely unremarkable. Initial laboratory testing, including blood cell count, electrolytes, thyroid panel, and pregnancy test, was normal. Urine drug toxicology screen was negative. The patient was admitted to the telemetry floor for syncope evaluation. How would you manage this case?

Case Review

This case revolves around the concept of syncope due to neurologic causes. Convulsive syncope should be considered in cases when a patient presents with sudden loss of consciousness, especially when no other etiologies can be identified. This is a typical case of seizure disorder, and the diagnosis usually does not require extensive workup. Brain imaging is required at the first unprovoked event or when hemorrhagic/traumatic, infectious, or demyelinating etiologies are considered. Electroencephalography (EEG) is diagnostic for seizure disorder. Antiepileptic drugs (AEDs) are not required after the first episode if high-risk factors are not present.

Case Discussion

A seizure disorder is a paroxysmal uncontrolled electrical activity of neurons that may involve a specific part of the brain or propagate to the entire cerebral cortex. Epilepsy consists of 2 events of unprovoked seizures. Tonic-clonic seizures, the most recognized type, can be focal (partial) or generalized depending on the loss of consciousness (generalized). Generalized seizure activity usually involves both cerebral hemispheres, and partial seizure activity arises in the temporal lobes.

Clinical Symptoms

A seizure disorder consists of stiffening and shaking movements of the body preceded by aura symptoms, which include abnormal auditory, tactile, or visual sensation. There can be a transient loss of consciousness based on the seizure type, followed by a postictal period of confusion or paralysis (Todd paralysis).

Management

The immediate management of seizure disorders should target stabilization of the airway, hemodynamic monitoring, and correction of reversible causes. Blood glucose, basic chemistry, liver function tests, drug toxicology screen, and AED and alcohol levels should be checked. A detailed evaluation of the sequence of events to identify provoked versus unprovoked etiology, family history of seizure disorder, risk factors for recurrence, and a history of childhood seizure disorder or of trauma should be obtained. Neuroimaging (brain CT or MRI) can be obtained in unprovoked seizure, trauma, focal neurologic deficit, or impaired mental status to identify structural causes. EEG should be obtained in unprovoked seizures or persistent altered mental status. Cerebrospinal fluid testing can be performed if infectious or inflammatory etiology is suspected. In cases of provoked seizures (metabolic, drug related, vasculitis, or infection), neuroimaging or EEG may not be needed if the cause is identified.

The management of a single unprovoked seizure disorder should be targeted to treat the underlying cause. AEDs should be initiated in cases of two or more unprovoked seizures or single unprovoked seizure with high-risk factors.

High-risk factors for recurrent seizure activity include the following:

- Age >65 years
- History of head trauma
- Partial seizure
- Postictal Todd paralysis
- Focal findings on EEG or brain MRI

Levetiracetam, lamotrigine, topiramate, valproic acid, and zonisamide are considered broad-spectrum agents that can be used to treat generalized and partial seizure disorders. Age, sex, comorbid conditions, and drug interactions should be considered before initiation. All patients should be screened for suicidal ideation. Patient should be educated about safety measures and avoid driving or other high-risk occupations.

Status epilepticus (SE) is persistent seizure activity with altered mentation lasting >5 minutes. Stability of the airway and measurement of vital signs and glucose levels should be performed immediately. Intramuscular midazolam or intravenous diazepam or lorazepam should be administered. Phenytoin or fosphenytoin should then be administered after the patient is stable, and in refractory cases, intubation and intravenous anesthetic agents are required. Continuous EEG monitoring is a part of SE management.

Key Points

- Convulsive syncope should be considered in syncope of unknown etiology if the cardiac and initial neurologic evaluations are negative.
- A detailed history of the sequence of events, family and social history, neuroimaging, and EEG are the cornerstones of the diagnostic process.
- Management requires identification of the etiology and its treatment in provoked cases.

4

10 Real Cases on Valvular Heart Disease: Diagnosis, Management, and Follow-Up

Nikhitha Mantri • Ayyadurai Pavanalingam • Marin Nicu

CASE 1

Management of Patent Foramen Ovale

A 26-year-old woman presented to the emergency department (ED) with chest pain for 1 day. The chest pain started suddenly, was nonradiating, and was associated with arm movement. She did house cleaning 1 day prior to presentation. The pain was not relieved by taking over-the-counter medication. She denied palpitations, dizziness, shortness of breath, and trauma. Her family history and social history were unremarkable. On presentation to the ED, her vital signs were stable. On physical examination, she did not have any significant findings except chest wall tenderness. Her ECG showed first-degree atrioventricular block. Initial laboratory findings were unremarkable. She was given analgesics. The patient was transferred to the telemetry floor, where an echocardiogram was performed, which showed a normal left ventricular ejection fraction with no wall motion or valvular abnormality and a small patent foramen ovale (PFO). How would you manage this case?

Case Review

This patient is a young asymptomatic woman who presented with musculoskeletal chest pain. Incidentally, she was noted to have a PFO, which is asymptomatic and does not require any treatment.

Case Discussion

PFO is an opening in the atrial wall at the location of the fossa ovalis that remains open beyond 1 year of life. After birth, when the pulmonary circulation develops, the foramen ovale closes due to the increase in left atrial pressures, which takes up to 1 year.

PFO is usually asymptomatic and is often found incidentally. However, it carries a risk of paradoxical embolism in high-risk patients. Some patients present with systemic embolism causing organ infarcts and even myocardial infarction.

The diagnostic test of choice is echocardiography. PFO can be detected using color flow Doppler, contrast echocardiography, and transmitral Doppler.

Management

Isolated PFO does not usually require any treatment unless it is associated with an unexplained neurologic event. Such conditions are treated with antiplatelet drugs and anticoagulation therapy. Percutaneous closure of the PFO is an option when there is contraindication to medical management and anticoagulant treatment, in the setting of paradoxical embolism or cryptogenic stroke. Surgical closure is indicated when the opening is >25 mm or when there is failure of a percutaneous device.

Key Points

- PFO is usually asymptomatic and is often found incidentally.
- Isolated PFO does not usually require any treatment unless it is associated with an unexplained neurologic event.

CASE 2

Management of Aortic Stenosis

A 78-year-old man with a medical history of hypertension and chronic obstructive pulmonary disease presented to the emergency department with worsening exercise tolerance for the past 6 months. He usually walks to his workplace, which is 6 blocks away from his home, but for the past few months, he has been barely able to walk for 2 to 3 blocks and has had to stop every 10 to 15 minutes to rest due to shortness of breath and chest tightness. On examination, the patient had a regular pulse and a blood pressure of 100/63 mm Hg and was afebrile. Examination revealed a thin body habitus. Cardiovascular examination revealed a hyperdynamic apical beat, systolic murmur in the aortic area, and carotid bruits. ECG showed normal sinus rhythm with left ventricular hypertrophy pattern. How would you manage this case?

Case Review

This case describes an elderly man with gradual worsening of cardiac symptoms. Examination is significant for wide pulse pressure and a systolic murmur best heard in the aortic area. ECG shows left ventricular hypertrophy (LVH). These factors point toward aortic stenosis (AS) as the most likely diagnosis in this patient. The etiology in this case is most likely calcification of the aortic valves. There are various manifestations of AS, which are described later in detail. Management includes both pharmacologic and surgical treatments depending on the degree of stenosis.

Case Discussion

AS is common in the elderly population. Etiology includes congenital valve abnormalities, calcification of the valve, trauma to the valve, and rheumatic heart disease, among other causes. The normal aortic valve area is approximately 3 to 4 cm^2 in adults. Usually patients are asymptomatic in their early stages. As the stenosis progresses, symptoms become more prominent, and the patient classically presents with syncope, angina, and heart failure.

Physical examination findings are often clues to the diagnosis, including single S_2 on auscultation and a systolic ejection murmur with radiation to carotid vessels.

Clinical Symptoms

Symptoms include dyspnea on exertion, dizziness, decreased exercise tolerance, syncope, chest pain or exertional angina, and palpitations.

Management

Echocardiogram is used to diagnose and evaluate the severity of AS. ECG usually shows LVH but is not diagnostic for AS. Doppler echocardiography can be used to assess the transaortic velocity, the left ventricular-aortic gradient, and the valve area.

There are various stages of severity of AS depending on the transvalvular aortic velocity. These include the following:

- Stage A: Includes maximum transvalvular aortic velocity <2 m/s. These patients are usually asymptomatic and have congenital aortic valve anomaly or aortic sclerosis or other risk factors for aortic valve disease such as smoking, male sex, metabolic syndrome, or old age.
- Stage B: Includes mild to moderate AS. These patients are usually symptomatic. The transvalvular aortic velocity for mild AS is 2.0 to 2.9 m/s, or the mean transvalvular pressure gradient is <20 mm Hg. For moderate AS, the transvalvular aortic velocity is 3.0 to 3.9 m/s, or the mean transvalvular pressure gradient is 20 to 39 mm Hg.
- Stage C: Includes severe valve obstruction but patients are asymptomatic. There is reduced leaflet motion and transvalvular aortic velocity ≥4 m/s. The aortic valve area is ≤1.0 cm^2.
- Stage D: Includes symptomatic patients with severe AS.

Treatment is usually valve replacement in patients who have severe AS. Balloon valvuloplasty is indicated in patients for palliative purposes. Pharmacologic management can be used in reducing symptoms but requires caution because even a mild imbalance can lead to hemodynamic instability. Diuretics, angiotensin-converting enzyme inhibitors, β-blockers, and sometimes digitalis can be used.

Key Points

- AS commonly presents with syncope, angina, or heart failure.
- Classification of AS is important because management varies based on stage.
- Definitive treatment includes aortic valve replacement.

CASE 3

Management of Mitral Stenosis

A 37-year-old woman was admitted to the telemetry floor for shortness of breath for 3 days. She immigrated from India recently and had a medical history significant for tuberculosis in childhood (completed treatment) and left chronic otitis media since childhood. She denied cough, fever, weight loss, or dizziness. She has 2 children and had no complications during pregnancy or in the postpartum period. The patient had stable vital signs.

On examination, she was found to have a grade 2/6 mid-diastolic murmur in the mitral area worsened by expiration and heard best in the left lateral position. The rest of the examination was normal. ECG showed normal sinus rhythm with bifid P waves. Pro-B-type natriuretic peptide was elevated. She was started on furosemide, and echocardiography was planned. How would you manage this patient?

Case Review

There are various causes of diastolic murmur in the mitral area. The murmur is typical for mitral stenosis (MS). This is a young patient with recurrent upper respiratory infection in childhood, who recently immigrated from a developing country and presented with a diastolic murmur in the mitral area. Childhood- or adult-onset rheumatic heart disease should be considered in this patient. MS can congenital or due to acquired calcification of the mitral valve. Most cases are secondary to rheumatic heart disease causing adhesions, thickening, and fibrosis of mitral leaflets, leading to MS. In this scenario, the patient appears to have congestive symptoms due to MS and will need further evaluation to assess the severity and determine further management.

Case Discussion

MS can be congenital or acquired, but most cases are attributed to rheumatic heart disease. The progression can be slow, but some patients can progress rapidly to heart failure, especially during pregnancy or when they have other significant comorbidities. The symptoms usually depend on the severity of stenosis.

Patients with MS are at a risk of developing atrial fibrillation secondary to atrial dilatation. This occurs due to increase in left atrial pressure due to mitral stenosis causing left atrial enlargement. This in turn causes stagnation of blood, leading to clot formation and the risk of thromboembolism. In addition, atrial fibrillation causes loss of atrial contraction, which is necessary for forward movement of blood, especially in patients with MS. Because these patients have a deformed mitral valve, it puts them at high risk for infective endocarditis.

Clinical Symptoms

MS can present with decreased exercise tolerance, dyspnea, orthopnea, fatigue, chest pain, palpitations (if atrial fibrillation develops), stroke (secondary to thromboembolism), hemoptysis (due to pulmonary vascular congestion), hoarseness (also known as Ortner syndrome and caused by compression of the recurrent laryngeal nerve by the enlarged left atrium), and even signs of right heart failure such as jugular venous distension, tender hepatomegaly, ascites, and pedal edema. Most of these symptoms are due to the backpressure caused by a narrowed mitral orifice, ultimately leading to pulmonary hypertension, increased right ventricular enlargement, tricuspid regurgitation, right atrial enlargement, and ultimately right heart failure.

On examination, MS patients can have diminished pulse volume. An irregularly irregular pulse will be present if the patient develops atrial fibrillation. Auscultation of the heart will reveal a loud S_1, but as the valves calcify, the S_1 diminishes in intensity. An opening snap is characteristic but may not be present in all cases. MS murmur is typically a low-pitched mid-diastolic murmur that is most prominent at the apex. Patients with pulmonary edema can have rales on lung examination. Signs of right-sided heart failure includes jugular venous distention, tender hepatomegaly, and pedal edema.

Management

Echocardiogram is diagnostic for MS. The degree of stenosis is essential for management. Pharmacologic management has limited role in mitral stenosis. β-Blockers and diuretics can be used with caution. Patients with atrial fibrillation will benefit from rate control medications and anticoagulation therapy.

MS is classified into various stages as shown in the table below.

Stage	Definition	Features	Symptoms
Stage A	Risk of MS	None	None
Stage B	Progressive MS	Increased transmitral flow velocities Mitral valve area (MVA) >1.5 cm²	None
Stage C	Asymptomatic, severe MS	MVA ≤1.5 cm² (MVA ≤1 cm² with severe MS)	None
Stage D	Symptomatic severe MS	MVA ≤1.5 cm² (MVA ≤1 cm² with severe MS)	Yes

Surgery is recommended for patients with stage D MS. Options include balloon valvuloplasty and commissurotomy.

Key Points

- MS is most commonly caused by rheumatic heart disease.
- The murmur typically present is a mid-diastolic murmur most prominent in the apex.
- There is limited role for pharmacologic management in MS.
- For patients with severe MS with symptoms, surgical therapy is warranted.

CASE 4

Management of Mitral Regurgitation

A 56-year-old man was admitted to the hospital with shortness of breath for 1 day. He was not able to lay flat and was feeling tired even while doing minimal activities. He recently experienced an anterior wall myocardial infarction (MI) for which he underwent percutaneous coronary intervention with stent placement and was discharged 2 days ago with medications. Prior to the MI, the patient was completely asymptomatic, and he has been compliant with medications. At presentation, the vital signs were stable. On physical examination, pulse was regular. Cardiac examination revealed a systolic murmur that was more prominent in the apex, radiating to the axilla. Lung examination showed bilateral crackles. ECG showed normal sinus rhythm with Q waves in inferior leads. Pro-B-type natriuretic peptide was elevated. He was planned for echocardiography. How would you manage this case?

Case Review

This patient has a systolic murmur in the apex radiating to axilla. Most likely, this patient developed acute mitral regurgitation (MR) after MI, which is a complication of MI. Such patients usually present with symptoms such as dyspnea, orthopnea, decreased exercise tolerance, and fatigue. In this case, the patient will need medications to reduce afterload to minimize symptoms due to MR. Diuretics can also be used for symptomatic relief. Surgical intervention is required in follow-up care.

Case Discussion

Acute MR is a common complication of MI. Other causes of MR include rheumatic heart disease, mitral valve prolapse, ischemic heart diseases, cardiomyopathy, infective endocarditis, and annular calcification. These patients are usually symptomatic due to the acute onset. Symptoms are partly due to impaired left ventricular (LV) function. The murmur is typically described as a high-pitched, blowing, holosystolic murmur best heard at the apex and radiating to axilla. S_1 may be diminished, S_2 is split, and a loud S_3 may be present. Mild MR is usually asymptomatic, but as the MR progresses in severity, LV failure occurs, causing pulmonary edema and, in turn, right heart failure.

Clinical Symptoms

These patients can present with dyspnea, fatigue, paroxysmal nocturnal dyspnea, orthopnea, chest pain, and palpitations.

Management

Echocardiogram and Doppler ultrasound are diagnostic and are useful for assessing severity of MR.

MR is classified into 4 stages, as shown in the following table.

Stage A	At risk of MR
Stage B	Asymptomatic with progressive MR
Stage C	Asymptomatic with severe MR; stage C1 (left ventricle [LV] or right ventricle [RV] remains compensated) or stage C2 (decompensation of LV or RV)
Stage D	Symptomatic with severe MR

Pharmacologic management includes use of drugs that reduce afterload (eg, angiotensin-converting enzyme inhibitors/angiotensin receptor blockers, nitrates, and antihypertensive drugs) and diuretics, which are used to maintain the forward cardiac output. β-Blockers are useful in patients who have concomitant LV dysfunction. Anticoagulation therapy should be considered when these patients develop atrial fibrillation.

Mitral valve surgery is indicated in symptomatic patients with LV ejection fraction (LVEF) >30% or in asymptomatic patients with LV dysfunction (ie, LV end-systolic diameter [LVESD] ≥45 mm and/or LVEF ≤60%). Surgery can also be considered in symptomatic patients who have severe LV dysfunction (LVEF <30% and/or LVESD >55 mm) and are refractory to pharmacologic therapy.

Key Points

- MR usually presents with a holosystolic murmur best heard at the apex.
- Medical therapy is directed at reducing afterload and thereby promoting forward flow of blood.

CASE 5

Management of Tricuspid Regurgitation

A 38-year-old woman with a history of smoking and intravenous drug use for the past 20 years presented to the hospital for central chest pain and high-grade fever that started 3 days ago. Chest pain was nonradiating and was associated with nonproductive cough. She had been treated for right-sided infective endocarditis last year and completed the 6-week antibiotic course. She has resumed doing recreational drugs over the past 2 months. In the emergency department, she was noted to have a temperature of 101°F with a heart rate of 98 bpm and blood pressure of 111/75 mm Hg. Physical examination revealed multiple track marks and tattoos over both upper extremities, right eye pterygium, and central obesity. Cardiac examination revealed a 2/6 holosystolic murmur at the left sternal border. Chest x-ray showed interstitial pattern edema bilaterally. ECG showed no abnormalities. Initial laboratory testing and blood cultures were sent, and she was transferred to the telemetry floor. How would you manage this case?

Case Review

This patient had a history of right-sided endocarditis and presented with a holosystolic murmur at the left sternal border and fever, which suggests tricuspid regurgitation (TR) and right-sided endocarditis. Prompt initiation of antibiotics with serial blood cultures should be performed. Echocardiogram should also be performed, along with daily ECGs to assess for valvular abscess.

Case Discussion

Isolated TR is not common. Etiologies for TR include rheumatic heart disease, infective endocarditis, carcinoid syndrome, congenital diseases such as Ebstein anomaly and endocardial cushion defects, and connective tissue disorders such as Marfan syndrome. Other causes include pulmonary hypertension, right ventricular failure, mitral stenosis or regurgitation, primary pulmonary disease, left-to-right shunts, Eisenmenger syndrome, pulmonary valve stenosis, and hyperthyroidism.

TR is usually asymptomatic, but in severe cases, patients will develop jugular venous distension, abdominal discomfort due to hepatomegaly, and bilateral lower extremity heaviness and swelling due to pedal edema. The murmur in TR is described as a holosystolic murmur heard best at the left lower sternal border. TR murmur is caused when there is movement of blood backward into the right atrium during systolic contraction. Mild to moderate TR is usually asymptomatic because the right atrium is very compliant. Severe TR causes right atrial dilatation and can cause signs of right heart failure such as jugular venous distension, ascites, tender hepatomegaly, and pedal edema. Chronic TR causes right ventricular volume overload, leading to right ventricular systolic dysfunction.

Clinical Symptoms

Symptoms depend on the underlying cause; for example, when a pulmonary disorder causes TR, patients can have symptoms such as shortness of breath, decreased exercise tolerance, or cough.

Management

Diagnosis is made by echocardiogram. The echocardiographic features indicative for severe TR include systolic flow reversal in the hepatic veins (specific for severe TR), 2-dimensional failure of coaptation or flail, large regurgitant jet on color Doppler, large flow convergence zone proximal to the valve, transtricuspid E wave dominant >1 cm/s, early peaking, and continuous wave Doppler of TR jet.

On the ECG, when right atrial enlargement is present, tall P waves are present, and when right ventricular enlargement is present, a tall R wave in lead V_1 >7 mm is present. X-ray of the chest can show right ventricular dilation and right atrial dilation. Lab tests may show some hepatic dysfunction in severe TR. Cardiac catheterization is indicated in severe TR for measurement of right-sided pressures.

Treatment of TR includes treating the underlying cause. Pharmacologic management includes use of diuretics; loop diuretics and aldosterone antagonists are typically used.

Annuloplasty or valve repair or replacement is the management of choice in patients with severe TR, in patients with symptoms despite medical treatment, or when there is moderate, progressive right ventricular enlargement or dysfunction.

Key Points

- TR is usually asymptomatic.
- Always look for underlying causes of TR because isolated primary TR is rare.
- Treatment includes managing the underlying cause. Initiate pharmacologic management with diuretics first, and if there is no response, then surgical treatment is indicated.

CASE 6

Management of Bicuspid Aortic Valve

A 43-year-old man was admitted to the telemetry floor with complaints of occasional chest pain on exertion and shortness of breath for 1 year, which have been gradually progressing for the past 3 months. He denied any other medical comorbidities except for well-controlled hyperthyroidism with medications. No social or family history was noted. The patient's vital signs were stable. On examination, the patient was found to have a diastolic murmur most prominent at the right upper sternal border. He had elevated jugular venous pressure and bilateral pedal edema. His ECG was unremarkable. Troponin and pro-B-type natriuretic peptide were elevated. On echocardiography, he was noticed to have reduced left ventricular ejection fraction and bicuspid aortic valve with no associated aortic valve abnormality. How would you manage this case?

Case Review

This case describes a middle-age patient with new-onset heart failure with reduced ejection fraction. He should be managed with diuretics and guideline-directed medical therapy for congestive heart failure. Evaluation for the cause of heart failure should be performed. He was also noticed to have a bicuspid aortic valve, which is not associated with the symptoms currently but will require surveillance of the patient and his family members.

Case Discussion

The normal aortic valve has 3 leaflets, which cause complete closure and opening of the aortic valve, allowing blood to flow in a forward direction. In a patient with a bicuspid aortic valve, imperfect opening and closure of the valve causes aortic insufficiency. The etiology of this disease is unknown. It is more common in males than females. These patients are known to have other cardiac conditions such as hypertension, abnormal coronaries, and aneurysms of the aorta.

This condition usually manifests at birth, but in most cases, these patients are asymptomatic and remain undiagnosed until later in life. Sometimes, the only evident sign is a murmur. It is uncommon for these patients to present with severe symptoms early in life or to develop heart failure.

Bicuspid aortic valves can develop stenosis due to calcium deposition or regurgitation due to backflow through the improperly closed valve. Chronic regurgitation can lead to left heart strain and failure. Patients with a bicuspid aortic valve also have a higher risk of infective endocarditis.

Clinical Symptoms

Symptoms include chest pain, shortness of breath, dizziness, loss of consciousness, and decreased exercise tolerance.

Management

Transthoracic echocardiography is the diagnostic test of choice for visualizing the anatomy. Additional information can be obtained by transesophageal echocardiography if coarctation of aorta, aneurysm of sinus of Valsalva, and patent ductus arteriosus are suspected. Other diagnostic tests include cardiac catheterization and cardiac CT if echocardiography remains unyielding.

Treatment should be directed to control hypertension. Pharmacologic management has limited role in treatment of bicuspid aortic valve disease.

Patients need monitoring with echocardiogram to prevent complications. Severe aortic stenosis requires annual surveillance echocardiography. For mild to moderate cases, follow-up every 3 to 5 years can be performed. First-degree relatives should be screened. Surgical management is indicated when the patient is symptomatic due to development of stenosis or regurgitation.

Key Points

- Bicuspid aortic valve is associated with complications such as aortic stenosis or regurgitation at comparatively younger age.
- Management consists of hypertension control and surveillance echocardiography for aortic valve complications.

CASE 7

Management of Aortic Regurgitation

A 68-year-old man was admitted to the telemetry floor for management of uncontrolled hypertension. He complained of headache and shortness of breath whenever his blood pressure got high. He was noted to have a blood pressure of 188/75 mm Hg that was equal in both arms. He stated that he takes all his medications, which include aspirin, hydrochloro-thiazide, losartan, and amlodipine. He denied nausea, vomiting, blurry vision, and neurologic deficit. His exercise tolerance was unlimited, but for the past 6 months, he started feeling shortness of breath even when walking 3 blocks. He denied smoking and other recreational drugs. On examination, the patient appeared thin, and pulsating neck veins were present. Cardiac examination revealed first and second heart sounds with a loud diastolic murmur in the right second intercostal space on the sternal border. Lung examination was clear. There were no other significant findings on examination. ECG showed left ventricular hypertrophy. How would you manage this case?

Case Review

This patient is an elderly man with risk factors including uncontrolled hypertension and decreased exercise tolerance. The patient was found to have a bounding pulse and high blood pressure with wide pulse pressure. Cardiac examination revealed a loud diastolic murmur in the aortic area on auscultation. All these findings suggest that the patient most likely has aortic regurgitation (AR). AR is common in the elderly population. Echocardiography can confirm the diagnosis, and treatment should be aimed at controlling the blood pressure. In patients with acute AR presenting with chest pain and uncontrolled blood pressure, aortic dissection should be ruled out.

Case Discussion

Acute AR is an emergent condition caused by aortic dissection or infective endocarditis. Chronic AR can be caused by various etiologies such as aortic root damage, rheumatic disease, bicuspid aortic valve, and valvular calcification. Damage to the aortic valve apparatus or aging causes AR, which in early stages can be mild. Over years, the left ventricle becomes hypertrophic to pump against the regurgitant volume, which may lead to ventricular dilation and left heart failure. These patients are initially asymptomatic for a long time until decompensation of the left ventricle occurs. These patients should be clinically monitored and should be treated before the decompensation phase begins. In contrast, acute AR presents with decompensated heart failure due to sudden onset of events.

Clinical Symptoms

Symptoms include exertional dyspnea, chest pain, orthopnea, paroxysmal nocturnal dyspnea, palpitations, dizziness, and syncope.

Clinical examination findings include diastolic murmur best heard over the right upper sternal border typically described as a crescendo-decrescendo murmur. Other examination findings include Corrigan pulse (rapid and forceful distension of the arterial pulse with a quick collapse), De Musset sign (bobbing of the head with each heartbeat), Muller sign (visible pulsations of the uvula), Quincke sign (capillary pulsations seen on light compression of the nail bed), Traube sign (systolic and diastolic sounds heard over the femoral artery), Duroziez sign (gradual pressure over the femoral artery leads to a systolic and diastolic bruit), and Hill sign (popliteal systolic blood pressure exceeding brachial systolic blood pressure by ≥60 mm Hg). These signs may or may not be present.

Management

Echocardiography (either transthoracic or transesophageal) is the diagnostic test of choice to assess the severity of valvular abnormality as well as the extent of heart failure. Cardiac magnetic resonance can be used if echocardiography results are suboptimal.

Staging of AR is shown in the following table.

Staging	Mild AR	Moderate AR	Severe AR
Parameters	Central jet, width <25% of left ventricular outflow tract (LVOT) Vena contracta <0.3 cm No or brief early diastolic flow reversal in descending aorta	Signs of AR > mild present but no criteria for severe AR	Central jet, width ≥65% of LVOT Vena contracta >0.6 cm

Patients with chronic AR should be monitored every year for progression of symptoms. Echocardiography can be repeated every 3 to 5 years for mild AR, every 1 to 2 years for moderate AR, and every 6 months to 1 year for severe AR.

Medical management is limited in this disease. Pharmacologic therapy includes use of diuretics, angiotensin-converting enzyme inhibitors or angiotensin II receptor blockers, β-blockers, mineralocorticoid receptor antagonists, and digoxin.

Aortic valve replacement is the treatment of choice for patients with severe symptomatic AR. Other indications include asymptomatic patients with chronic severe AR and evidence of left ventricular systolic dysfunction with an ejection fraction of <50%, asymptomatic patients with chronic severe AR with a normal left ventricular ejection fraction (≥50%) but with an end-systolic dimension >50 mm, and patients with severe AR undergoing cardiac surgery for other indications.

Acute AR is an emergent situation, and aortic valve surgery should be performed immediately.

Key Points

- Acute AR is an emergent condition and requires immediate valve replacement.
- Chronic aortic regurgitation usually has a long course over years, ending eventually in heart failure. These patients should be monitored periodically for worsening of symptoms.
- Surgery is the management of choice.

CASE 8

Management of Pulmonary Stenosis

A 23-year-old woman was admitted to the telemetry floor for palpitations of 3 hours in duration. She started having symptoms while at work. She had no history of cardiovascular disease and can perform unlimited exercise. She denied any toxic habits and family history of heart disease. Her vitals were stable. Physical examination revealed a thin girl. Lung auscultation revealed bilateral rhonchi. Cardiac examination revealed a normal S_1 and a split S_2. A grade 2/6 ejection systolic murmur was present and most audible at the left upper sternal border. ECG showed normal sinus rhythm. How would you manage this case?

Case Review

This otherwise healthy patient with palpitations was found to have an incidental finding of a cardiac murmur on auscultation. She is completely asymptomatic and actively participates in sports. An ejection systolic murmur best heard at the left upper sternal border is a classic presentation of pulmonary stenosis. An echocardiogram can be obtained to assess the severity of stenosis. There is very little role of pharmacologic management in pulmonary stenosis. This patient should be monitored by a telemetry monitor for any arrythmia.

Case Discussion

The etiology of pulmonary stenosis is most often congenital. It can present as isolated pulmonary stenosis or can be a part of syndromes such as tetralogy of Fallot, Noonan syndrome, and congenital rubella syndrome. The pulmonary valve can be stenotic or atretic, causing narrowing of the ostia and turbulent blood flow through the valves. Rarely, the stenosis can be due to acquired conditions such as rheumatic fever and carcinoid or collagen vascular diseases. These patients are usually asymptomatic; murmur on auscultation is usually an incidental finding in most cases. Pulmonary stenosis can also be supravalvular, valvular, or subvalvular. These patients may have a coexisting patent foramen ovale or ventricular septal defect. The pulmonary artery is dilated in most cases. Over time, the right ventricle becomes hypertrophied as it pumps against the stenotic valve, leading to right heart dilation and failure. This ultimately progresses to cause tricuspid regurgitation, right atrial dilation, and signs of right heart failure, including jugular venous distention, tender hepatomegaly, ascites, and pedal edema. Presence of concomitant ventricular or atrial septal defect or patent foramen ovale leads to a right-to-left shunt, causing cyanosis.

Clinical Symptoms

These patients are usually asymptomatic. When symptomatic, patients can present with exertional dyspnea, shortness of breath, cyanosis, chest pain, palpitations, and lower extremity swelling when right heart failure occurs.

On clinical examination, the murmur in PS is an ejection systolic murmur present in the left upper sternal border that radiates to the axilla, the infraclavicular area, or the back.

Management

Echocardiography (Doppler) is the diagnostic test of choice. ECG can show right ventricular or atrial hypertrophy. The severity is classified based on the pulmonary valvular gradient, as shown in the table below.

Stage	Gradient
Trivial	<25 mm Hg
Mild	25-49 mm Hg
Moderate	50-79 mm Hg
Severe	>80 mm Hg

Cardiac catheterization is useful in cases where echocardiography cannot provide the diagnosis. Pharmacologic therapy has a very limited role in the treatment of pulmonary stenosis. Patients who have moderate or severe pulmonary stenosis will need balloon valvuloplasty or surgical intervention to relieve the stenosis.

Key Points

- Pulmonary stenosis is mostly associated with other congenital anomalies.
- Valvuloplasty is the treatment of choice if patients present with severe symptomatic pulmonary stenosis or if they develop right heart failure.

CASE 9

Management of Late-Life Complications of Coarctation of Aorta

A 32-year-old man presented to the emergency department (ED) with a complaint of shortness of breath for the past 6 months that had progressed to an extent that he was not able to walk a few steps. He had been following up with his primary care physician for hypertension, and despite taking 3 antihypertensive medications (amlodipine, hydrochlorothiazide, and losartan), his blood pressure (BP) remained uncontrolled. His medical history consisted of aortic coarctation that was repaired in childhood, after which he never followed up with a cardiologist. He did not have any toxic habits and denied family history of cardiac disease. In the ED, his vital signs were noted as BP of 170/95 mm Hg, heart rate of 80 bpm, respiratory rate of 18 breath/min, and oxygen saturation of 98% on room air. On physical examination, the patient was found to have bilateral rales with elevated jugular venous pressure and systolic murmur in the aortic area, and faint femoral pulses palpated bilaterally with radiofemoral delay. ECG showed normal sinus rhythm with left ventricular hypertrophy. Chest x-ray showed interstitial edema. Pro-B-type natriuretic peptide was elevated. How would you manage this case?

Case Review

This case deals with the late-life complications after repair of coarctation of the aorta. In this particular case, the patient presented with symptoms of pulmonary edema in the setting of uncontrolled hypertension. BP control is the cornerstone of treatment. Echocardiography can be used to diagnose underlying heart failure, valvular heart disease, or recoarctation of aorta. Aortic dissection should also be considered in the evaluation process.

Case Discussion

Aortic coarctation is a narrowing usually beyond the origin of the left subclavian artery. Patients with repaired coarctation can present with late-life complications, including malignant hypertension, aortic aneurysms, premature coronary artery disease, aortic valve problems, and cerebral aneurysms. Women are also at risk of pregnancy-related complications. Recoarctation can also occur after surgery or angioplasty. Diagnosis is usually made by clinical findings of delay in upper and lower extremity pulses and supportive findings such as a chest x-ray showing rib notching and a figure 3 sign (dilatation of aorta above and below coarctation). A transthoracic echocardiography is used to assess the severity of coarctation using the suprasternal view. Doppler can be used to assess the gradient of severity and to identify the diastolic runoff at the coarctation site. CT angiography or cardiac catheterization is used in further assessment of anatomy and associated anomalies.

Clinical Symptoms

Symptoms include systemic hypertension, intermittent claudication, decreased exercise tolerance, and headache.

Management

Transcatheter intervention (ie, balloon angioplasty with or without stent placement) is indicated in patients with recoarctation with a gradient of >20 mm Hg, imaging evidence of collateral circulation, or development of hypertension as a consequence of recoarctation. For patients with concomitant arch hypoplasia, long recoarctation segment, or aortic aneurysm, surgical repair is preferred.

Pharmacologic management involves hypertension control using β-blockers, angiotensin-converting enzyme inhibitors, angiotensin receptor blockers, or calcium channel blockers.

There is no indication for infective endocarditis (IE) prophylaxis after surgical repair unless there is a history of IE.

All patients should be followed by a cardiologist on an annual basis, with surveillance imaging (CT/MRI) to evaluate the aortic root performed every 3 to 5 years.

Key Points

- Patients with repaired coarctation of aorta can present with late-life complications such as malignant hypertension, aortic valve problems, and cerebral aneurysms.
- All patients should have lifelong congenital cardiology follow-up and surveillance imaging.
- Medical management includes control of hypertension.

CASE 10

Management of Tricuspid Stenosis

A 23-year-old Hispanic man was admitted to the telemetry floor for progressive worsening of shortness of breath for 4 months that has recently worsened significantly. He was previously able to walk 3 or 4 blocks without difficulty, but this deteriorated to feeling short of breath with daily activities. He denied any history of syncope, lightheadedness, dizziness, palpitations, leg swelling, chest pain, cough, or fever. His medical conditions included hypertension, hyperlipidemia, obesity, heart failure, and aortic stenosis. His family history was unremarkable for any cardiac condition. He did not remember his medications. He denied any history of smoking or alcohol use or any other recreational drug habits. He works in an office and lives with his family at home. On physical examination, his vital signs were stable. He was obese with no signs of distress. Focused cardiovascular examination showed palpable and equal pulses in all extremities, and elevated jugular venous pulsations were seen. Pulmonary examination showed bilateral rales. Cardiac examination showed regular S_1 and S_2 with a 3/6 systolic murmur at the left lower sternal border in the third intercostal space radiating to carotids. The rest of the physical examination was unremarkable. ECG showed sinus rhythm with intraventricular conduction delay. On laboratory testing, pro-B-type natriuretic peptide was elevated. Transthoracic echocardiogram showed a fibrocalcific aortic valve with moderate aortic stenosis. Transesophageal echocardiography (TEE) was performed to further evaluate an aortic valve that showed moderate aortic stenosis with bicuspid aortic valve. There was mild apical displacement of tricuspid valve leaflets with suspicion of Ebstein anomaly. How would you address this patient's TEE findings?

Case Review

This case describes the management of tricuspid stenosis (TS). The patient presented with typical heart failure symptoms, but the TEE showed suspicion of tricuspid atresia. His symptoms cannot be completely attributed to aortic stenosis, and thus, cardiac MRI should be performed to further assess the right ventricle structure. Currently, the patient can be managed with diuretics until the diagnosis is established. Ebstein anomaly consists of apical displacement of the tricuspid valve, leading to arterialization of the right ventricle.

Case Discussion

Isolated TS is rare and is usually associated with other valvular lesions. There are many causes of TS, such as rheumatic heart disease (most common), carcinoid syndrome, congenital atresia or stenosis, tumors of the right heart, infective endocarditis, systemic lupus erythematosus, and hypereosinophilic syndrome. Ebstein anomaly is a rare cause of TS that can be associated with arrythmia and right heart failure. Once stenosis of the tricuspid valve develops, as a result of narrowing of the orifice, there will be gradual dilation of the right atrium and systemic venous congestion leading to jugular venous distention, tender hepatomegaly, ascites, and pedal edema leading to right heart failure. However, these symptoms rarely occur. In certain cases, when the stenosis is severe enough to obstruct forward flow of the blood causing decreased cardiac output, patients can present with fatigue, exertional dyspnea, and dizziness.

Physical examination may reveal an opening snap and diastolic murmur at the left lower sternal border that is usually audible when isolated TS is present. When TS is associated with other valvular diseases, the opening snap may be overlapped by other murmurs.

Management

Diagnosis is usually made by transthoracic echocardiography, which can aid in delineating the etiology of TS. Doppler echocardiography can be used to determine the flow gradient. Cardiac catheterization can be used to determine the severity of TS. The presence of concomitant tricuspid regurgitation can change the management.

ECG is usually nondiagnostic but can sometimes show tall P waves indicating right atrial enlargement. Atrial fibrillation is an associated arrythmia. Ebstein anomaly is associated with Wolff-Parkinson-White pattern on the ECG.

A peak flow velocity of >1 m/s during inspiration, a valve area of ≤1 cm², and an inflow time-velocity integral >60 cm indicate hemodynamically significant TS.

Pharmacologic management involves the use of loop diuretics and aldosterone antagonists to reduce congestion. In severe TS, surgical valve repair or replacement or balloon valvotomy is indicated. If patient develops atrial fibrillation, use of rate or rhythm control medications and anticoagulation is advisable.

Key Points

- TS rarely occurs as an isolated valvular disease. The most common etiology is rheumatic heart disease; however, other underlying causes such as congenital heart disease can be present.
- Treatment includes use of diuretics and, if indicated, valve surgery.

5

10 Real Cases on Acute Heart Failure Syndrome: Diagnosis, Management, and Follow-Up

Swathi Roy • Gayathri Kamalakkannan

CASE 1

Diagnosis and Management of New-Onset Heart Failure With Reduced Ejection Fraction

A 54-year-old woman presented to the telemetry floor with shortness of breath (SOB) for 4 months that progressed to an extent that she was unable to perform daily activities. She also used 3 pillows to sleep and often woke up from sleep due to difficulty catching her breath. Her medical history included hypertension, dyslipidemia, diabetes mellitus, and history of triple bypass surgery 4 years ago. Her current home medications included aspirin, atorvastatin, amlodipine, and metformin. No significant social or family history was noted. Her vital signs were stable. Physical examination showed bilateral diffuse crackles in lungs, elevated jugular venous pressure, and 2+ pitting lower extremity edema. ECG showed normal sinus rhythm with left ventricular hypertrophy. Chest x-ray showed vascular congestion. Laboratory results showed a pro-B-type natriuretic peptide (pro-BNP) level of 874 pg/mL and troponin level of 0.22 ng/mL. Thyroid panel was normal. An echocardiogram demonstrated systolic dysfunction, mild mitral regurgitation, a dilated left atrium, and an ejection fraction (EF) of 33%. How would you manage this case?

Case Review

In this case, a patient with known history of coronary artery disease presented with worsening of shortness of breath with lower extremity edema and jugular venous distension along with crackles in the lung. The sign and symptoms along with labs and imaging findings point to diagnosis of heart failure with reduced EF (HFrEF). She should be treated with diuretics and guideline-directed medical therapy for congestive heart failure (CHF). Telemetry monitoring for arrythmia should be performed, especially with structural heart disease. Electrolyte and urine output monitoring should be continued.

Case Discussion

In the initial evaluation of patients who present with signs and symptoms of heart failure, pro-BNP level measurement may be used as both a diagnostic and prognostic tool. Based on left ventricular EF (LVEF), heart failure is classified into heart failure with preserved EF (HFpEF) if LVEF is >50%, HFrEF if LVEF is <40%, and heart failure with mid-range EF (HFmEF) if LVEF is 40% to 50%. All patients with symptomatic heart failure should be started on an angiotensin-converting enzyme (ACE) inhibitor (or angiotensin receptor blocker if ACE inhibitor is not tolerated) and β-blocker, as appropriate. In addition, in patients with New York Heart Association functional classes II through IV, an aldosterone antagonist should be prescribed. In African American patients, hydralazine and nitrates should be added. Recent recommendations also recommend starting an angiotensin receptor-neprilysin inhibitor (ARNI) in patients who are symptomatic on ACE inhibitors.

Alternatively, ARNI could be started instead of ACE inhibitors or ARBs. Loop diuretics may be added to relieve symptoms of congestion. They help in improving quality of life by decreasing fluid retention and thus relieving symptoms but have shown no mortality benefit. Medications should be started at low doses and gradually titrated up to recommended target doses. Digoxin can also be considered in patients who are symptomatic despite being on ACE inhibitors/ARBs, β-blockers, and mineralocorticoid receptor antagonists (MRAs) to reduce the risk of hospitalization. Ischemia evaluation can be considered in patients with angina symptoms.

In patients who can tolerate neither ACE inhibitors nor ARBs (or for patients in whom they are contraindicated), the combination of hydralazine and isosorbide dinitrate may be considered.

Early follow-up within a week is recommended for all patients with heart failure after hospital discharge. Educating patients about dietary habits, adherence to medications, and lifestyle modification is an important component of managing heart failure.

Key Points

- Diagnosis of heart failure is challenging, with history and physical examination playing a key role in diagnosis, followed by echocardiography.
- Symptoms such as orthopnea and paroxysmal nocturnal dyspnea are more specific to the diagnosis of heart failure.
- Diuretics are recommended to improve symptoms and exercise capacity in patients with signs or symptoms of CHF.
- Early follow-up within a week is recommended for all patients with heart failure after hospital discharge.
- Educating patients about dietary habits, adherence to medications, and lifestyle modification is an important component of managing heart failure.

CASE 2

Management of Ischemic Cardiomyopathy

A 56-year-old man presented to emergency department with complaints of shortness of breath that have progressively worsened over the past 2 months. At baseline, on a flat surface, he could walk 6 blocks, but at presentation, this decreased to 2 blocks. He stated that he has gained 10 pounds and has increased swelling of his feet. His medical history included asthma, hypertension, dyslipidemia, and obesity. He is a smoker and works as an office manager. He had seen his primary care physician who suggested that his asthma might be causing his symptoms, and he was asked to take albuterol as needed, which did not improve his symptoms. He appeared to be in mild distress with stable vital signs and had jugular venous distension. He also had bibasilar crackles in the lungs, an S_3 heart sound, and bilateral pedal edema. His ECG showed Q waves, nonspecific ST changes, and left ventricular hypertrophy. His troponin levels were elevated but not trending up. Pro-B-type natriuretic peptide was 680 pg/dL. He was started on intravenous furosemide and noninvasive positive-pressure ventilation. Th next day, his echocardiography showed a left ventricular ejection fraction (LVEF) of 32% and regional wall motion abnormalities. How would you manage this case?

Case Review

This patient had suspected ischemic cardiomyopathy. He underwent coronary angiography and was found to have a mid-left anterior descending artery lesion for which percutaneous coronary intervention (PCI) was performed. The patient was started on dual antiplatelet therapy along with a statin. In addition, he was discharged on an angiotensin-converting enzyme inhibitor (ACEI), mineralocorticoid receptor antagonist (MRA), and β-blocker and advised to follow up in the cardiology clinic within a week. He was also provided with an external wearable defibrillator.

Case Discussion

The etiology of heart failure with reduced ejection fraction includes coronary artery disease (CAD), valvular heart disease, arrhythmias, and high-output heart failure. Myocardial ischemia is associated with cardiac remodeling, leading to progressive changes in shape and size of the heart. Patients with ischemia as an underlying etiology of heart failure can present with angina or its equivalents, along with ischemic ECG changes. Echocardiography can help to determine the etiology, such as valvular disorders or wall motion abnormities. Patients with angina symptoms or hemodynamic instability in association with electrical instability should be assessed for CAD by coronary angiogram. Cardiac catheterization is also indicated if high-risk factors for CAD such as dyslipidemia, cocaine abuse, and obesity are present with positive stress testing. PCI should be performed if any evidence of coronary occlusion is present. In such cases, dual antiplatelet therapy should be continued along with guideline-directed medical therapy (GDMT) for heart failure. Ischemic cardiomyopathy is associated with higher risk of fatal ventricular arrhythmias, and in order to prevent sudden cardiac death, an external wearable defibrillator is advised until improvement in ejection fraction is seen. An implantable cardioverter-defibrillator should be considered after PCI if ejection fraction does not improve after 3 months of optimized GDMT. GDMT consists of ACEIs/angiotensin receptor blockers, β-blockers, MRAs, and angiotensin receptor-neprilysin inhibitors, with patient education and lifestyle modifications to control the risk factors.

Key Points

- Ischemic cardiomyopathy is a major cause of heart failure and should be evaluated in the setting of angina symptoms.
- Management should be targeted to revascularize the ischemic myocardium and should also include GDMT.

CASE 3

Management of Tachycardia-Induced Cardiomyopathy

A 62-year-old woman presented to the emergency department (ED) with sudden onset of palpitations that started while gardening. She had been having similar episodes for the past 4 to 5 months that lasted for few minutes and resolved on their own. Recently, she started having shortness of breath on exertion, which had been progressively worsening. She had become unable to lay flat, and her exercise tolerance had decreased from 5 blocks to 1 block. She stated that she drinks 5 cups of caffeinated beverages daily. She denied having any chest pain, dizziness, or syncope. Her medical comorbidities included hypertension and anxiety disorder. She denied taking any over-the-counter supplements or drugs. She had no family history of heart disease and had never smoked or used any recreational drugs. In the ED, her vital signs showed a blood pressure of 140/84 mm Hg and a pulse of 180 bpm. On physical examination, she was in mild respiratory distress with jugular venous distension. On lung examination, she had coarse bibasilar crackles bilaterally. No pedal edema was noted. Chest radiography showed pulmonary vascular congestion and right basal infiltrates. Pro-B-type natriuretic peptide and troponin levels were elevated but not trending up. Her ECG showed supraventricular tachycardia, no P waves, and narrow QRS complexes. To determine the underlying rhythm, a vagal maneuver was attempted that slowed down the rate, and the rhythm was determined as atrial flutter. She was admitted to the telemetry floor, where rate was controlled by metoprolol. Echocardiography showed a left ventricular ejection fraction of 30% with no wall motion or valvular abnormalities. She underwent catheter ablation of the ectopic focus and was converted to sinus rhythm. She was discharged and was seen in clinic in 2 weeks later, where repeat echocardiography showed an ejection fraction of 62% with cardiac dilatation.

Case Review

The patient presented with palpitations and acute onset of dyspnea and was found to have tachycardia; in addition, the ECG showed atrial flutter with rapid ventricular rate. Her cardiomyopathy is most likely tachycardia induced. With rate control or cardioversion, cardiomyopathy can be reversed, thus treating the underlying cause.

Case Discussion

Tachycardia-induced cardiomyopathy is a reversible form of cardiomyopathy that can manifest from months to years after tachycardia onset. It is usually observed in supraventricular tachycardia and can be precipitated by a high burden of premature ventricular contractions, such as bigeminy. It is highly dependent on the ventricular rate, but no cutoff rates have been established. The hallmark feature is restoration of rate and rhythm, leading to normalization of left ventricular function and ejection fraction. The main principle in management of tachycardia-induced cardiomyopathy causing heart failure with reduced ejection fraction is heart rate normalization, either with rate or rhythm control. The decision to pursue an ischemic workup should be based on clinical suspicion and risk factors, but in general, it is not necessary.

Treatment of the underlying etiology is the cornerstone of therapy. There may be no underlying structural heart disease primarily responsible for the cardiac dysfunction. Thyroid function should be tested, and urine drug screen should be performed. Caffeine intake and other caffeinated beverages should be restricted. Long-term treatment may include diuretics such as furosemide, angiotensin-converting enzyme inhibitors, β-blockers, and, in some cases, ablation. Usually ejection fraction improves as early as 1 week after treatment, and complete resolution occurs in 4 to 6 weeks.

Key Points

- Tachycardia-induced cardiomyopathy is a reversible form of cardiomyopathy associated with no structural heart disease.
- Controlling the tachycardia leads to improvement in ejection fraction.
- Treatment of the underlying etiology is the cornerstone of therapy.

CASE 4

Heart Failure With Reduced Ejection Fraction and Use of Diuretics

A 70-year-old man presented to the emergency department (ED) with complaints of dyspnea for 4 weeks, which had been progressively worsening, limiting his exercise tolerance from 4 blocks to half a block. He did not complain of chest pain or palpitations. His medical history included hypertension, paroxysmal atrial fibrillation, coronary artery disease status post percutaneous coronary intervention (PCI) to mid-left anterior descending artery (LAD) 2 years ago, and heart failure with reduced ejection fraction (HFrEF) (left ventricular ejection fraction, 40%). His medications included furosemide 40 mg once a day, metoprolol succinate, aspirin, dabigatran, and atorvastatin. He admitted to smoking crack cocaine and drinking alcohol every day. In the ED, vital signs were stable, with a blood pressure of 110/70 mm Hg, pulse of 70 bpm, and respiratory rate of 20 breath/min. On physical examination, the patient was in respiratory distress using accessory muscles of respiration. He had bibasilar crackles on examination, no murmurs, loud S_3, abdominal distension, and positive hepatojugular reflex. He also had pedal edema extending to mid-thigh. His ECG showed left ventricular hypertrophy with left axis deviation. Chest radiography showed bilateral congestion. Pro-B-type natriuretic peptide and troponin levels were elevated but not trending up. His creatinine was elevated from baseline. He was initiated on intravenous furosemide and bilevel positive airway pressure therapy. How would you manage the case on the telemetry floor?

Case Review

This patient with known HFrEF who has been on diuretic therapy appears to be experiencing an exacerbation of heart failure. He is wet and warm in terms of volume status and perfusion and hence can be treated with diuretics. His urine output should be strictly quantified along with daily weight and monitoring of electrolytes. Diuretics should be titrated based on volume status and improvement in clinical status. Creatinine usually improves with improvement in renal congestion. Education regarding avoiding cocaine and remaining adherent to the medication regimen should be provided.

Case Discussion

The goal of acute heart failure exacerbation management is not only to excrete salt, but also to maintain a net negative water balance. First and foremost, the patient's adherence to diet and medications needs to be assessed. Elderly patients often take over-the-counter nonsteroidal anti-inflammatory drugs and should be educated to avoid such medications. The cornerstone of treatment of acute heart failure syndrome (AHFS) is diuretics, and the most commonly used agents are loop diuretics due to their greater efficacy. Furosemide, bumetanide, and torsemide are loop diuretics used for diuresis in routine practice. AHFS management can also be guided by the following algorithm using volume and perfusion status.

Warm and Dry (Euvolemic)	**Warm and Wet** (Hypervolemic) Initiate furosemide
Cold and Wet (Hypervolemic) Initiate furosemide	**Cold and Dry** (Cardiogenic shock) Initiate inotropes

In AHFS, furosemide can be initiated either as bolus or continuous infusion to achieve target negative water balance of 3 to 5 L. The dose of intravenous furosemide can be roughly estimated by using a dose 2.5 times higher than home dose. Clinical examination should be performed and urine output and daily weight should be strictly monitored, and diuretic dose can be adjusted based on the results. Laboratory parameters such as hematocrit, blood urea nitrogen, and bicarbonate levels can be used to assess diuresis. Renal function can initially fluctuate and then stabilize after continued diuresis, but excessive diuresis can lead to dehydration. Dehydration should be monitored by performing a clinical examination. In cases where optimal diuresis cannot be achieved even with maximum doses of a single loop diuretic, sequential blockade can be initiated using thiazide diuretics. If sequential diuresis remains unsuccessful, ultrafiltration can be used. During the diuresis phase, electrolytes such as potassium and magnesium should be adequately replenished to avoid fatal arrythmias.

Key Points

- AHFS is managed by diuresis using loop diuretics guided by clinical examination, urine output, and daily weight monitoring.
- Adequate euvolemia should be achieved to avoid recurrent exacerbation, and the patient should be educated regarding medication adherence, dietary changes, and fluid restriction.

CASE 5

Heart Failure With Reduced Ejection Fraction: Use of Inotropes

A 76-year-old man was admitted to the telemetry floor after 2 episodes of near-syncope. He further stated that he was short of breath on walking less than half a block. The shortness of breath had progressively worsened to the point that he was unable to lay down flat and had to sleep propped up on his bed. He denied chest pain, palpitations, and dizziness. His medical history included hypertension, coronary artery disease (status post coronary artery bypass graft [CABG] 3 years ago), heart failure with reduced ejection fraction (ejection fraction, 15%; global hypokinesia) status post automated implantable cardioverter-defibrillator (AICD), New York Heart Association (NYHA) class IV, recently diagnosed advanced pancreatic cancer, asthma/chronic obstructive pulmonary disease (never intubated), and dyslipidemia.

He was adherent to his medications, which included metoprolol succinate 200 mg once daily, furosemide 80 mg twice daily, atorvastatin 40 mg once daily at night, aspirin 81 mg once daily, lisinopril 20 mg once daily, and spironolactone 50 mg once daily. He had also been following a low-salt diet and avoided any salty food. He stopped smoking 8 years ago and denied alcohol and drug abuse. He has had multiple admissions in the past year for heart failure despite being adherent to medications, diet and fluid restriction, and lifestyle management. On physical examination, he was hypotensive with a blood pressure of 84/74 mm Hg, was afebrile, and had a pulse of 96 bpm. His extremities were cold. He was in respiratory distress and using accessory muscles of respiration, and he had jugular venous distension to 12 cm H_2O, bilateral crackles in all lung fields, and diffuse wheezing. He also had 2+ pitting lower extremity edema. He had an S_3 gallop and no murmurs or abdominal distension but had tender hepatomegaly. ECG showed a paced heart rate of 72 bpm, and chest x-ray showed bilateral pleural effusions and cardiomegaly. His white blood cell count and comprehensive metabolic panel were within normal limits except for creatinine of 2.4 mg/dL (baseline, 1.2 mg/dL). He was started on dobutamine and furosemide drip with strict urine output monitoring and was transferred to a cardiac intensive care unit. The echocardiography showed ejection fraction of 12% and minimal pericardial effusion. He was continued on sequential diuresis; however, he continued to have a net positive water balance. His renal function showed a creatinine bump to 4.8 mg/dL. After this, the patient was started on low-dose dopamine. Over the course of a few days, he developed a net negative water balance of 3 L/d and his creatinine returned to baseline. Multiple attempts to wean him off inotropes remained unsuccessful. A palliative care team was consulted to discuss goals of care. He wished for home hospice care. He was continued on dobutamine and planned for discharge to home hospice.

Case Review

This patient has a history of ischemic cardiomyopathy (NYHA class IV) with CABG/AICD and has had frequent admissions in the past year for heart failure despite compliance with maximal medical therapy and adherence to diet and fluid restriction. He presented with signs and symptoms of heart failure. On examination, he was classified as "wet and cold," and hence, he was started on inotropes, which could not be tapered off in the hospital. The patient was discharged to home hospice on long-term inotropic therapy.

Case Discussion

Cardiogenic shock is defined as a sustained systolic blood pressure <90 mm Hg or mean arterial pressure (MAP) <65 mm Hg for >30 minutes or the use of inotropes is required to achieve this. Patients with cardiogenic shock usually present with pulmonary congestion, cold clammy skin, decreased urine output, and altered mental state. Vasotropes and inotropes are the main therapies in managing cardiogenic shock. In cases refractory to diuretics, in which there is worsening of cardiorenal syndrome, inotropes transiently allow a reduction in right atrial and renal venous pressures to achieve effective diuresis and symptom relief. Inotropes not only improve the contractility of the myocardium but also affect the heart rate and peripheral vascular resistance. Inotropic agents increase myocardial contractility, thereby increasing cardiac output, whereas vasopressors/vasotropes increase the blood pressure. In general, inotropes should be used at the lowest dose required to achieve clinical effect. The most commonly used medications are:

- Epinephrine, norepinephrine, dopamine, and dobutamine, which primarily act on α and/or β receptors and/or D_1/D_2 receptors
- Phosphodiesterase inhibitors: milrinone and amrinone
- Calcium sensitizers
- Vasopressin

α-Adrenergic activity constricts peripheral arterioles, increasing systemic vascular resistance (SVR), which reduces stroke volume. The overall effect is a small net change in cardiac output, but it raises blood pressure and shifts blood away from the periphery and toward the coronary arteries and brain. Norepinephrine increases cardiac output and mixed venous oxygen without increasing heart rate, making it pressor of choice. Epinephrine acts on both alpha and beta. An increase in heart rate causes increased oxygen consumption and hence epinephrine may not be the best option. As a vasopressor and as an inotrope, it is usually considered a second-line agent. Dopamine is an α- and β-adrenergic agonist that also stimulates dopaminergic receptors D_1 and D_2. It is used as an inotrope in low cardiac output states, where it increases MAP primarily by increasing cardiac index with minimal effects on SVR. Dobutamine has predominant β-adrenergic activity and only limited α-adrenergic activity. Given its $β_1$ receptor–mediated positive inotropic action and $β_2$ receptor–mediated vasodilatory action, dobutamine increases cardiac output and decreases systemic and pulmonary vascular resistance. Dobutamine is the preferred vasoactive agent to treat cardiogenic shock in patients with low output and increased afterload. Vasopressin V_1 receptor stimulation in smooth muscle wall mediates vasoconstriction, whereas V_2 receptor activation mediates water reabsorption in the collecting duct. These effects tend to cause an increase in SVR. Milrinone causes cardiac inotropy and arteriolar and venous dilation. The net result is increased cardiac index. It is used in refractory cardiogenic shock.

Key Points

- Cardiogenic shock with organ dysfunction is a Class I indication for temporary inotropic therapy to support perfusion while other strategies such as a ventricular assist device or cardiac transplant are being sought.
- Treatment with inotropes is a Class IIB indication as a purely palliative measure. It can be prescribed on a long-term basis as outpatient inotrope infusions.

CASE 6

Heart Failure With Preserved Ejection Fraction and Valvular Heart Disease

A 78-year-old man presented with complaints of gradual onset of shortness of breath that had progressively worsened over the past 5 to 6 weeks to the extent that the patient was unable to lie down flat. He was fatigued throughout the day and had difficulty concentrating and performing activities of daily living. He had shortness of breath for the past year. He also complained of occasional chest pain on exertion over the past few days that lasted for a few minutes and subsided with rest. His medical comorbidities included uncontrolled diabetes, uncontrolled hypertension, dyslipidemia, and mild aortic stenosis diagnosed 3 years ago. He was a current smoker and smoked 15 to 20 cigarettes per day for 56 years. On clinical examination, he had a crescendo-decrescendo systolic murmur along the left sternal border radiating to the upper right sternal border and into the carotid arteries and a single S_2. He also had crackles throughout the lung field. His chest x-ray showed marked cardiomegaly and vascular congestion, and ECG showed left ventricular hypertrophy with repolarization abnormalities. On echocardiography, there was calcification of aortic valve leaflets with reduced leaflet mobility. Doppler evaluation showed a mean gradient of 44 mm Hg and aortic valve area of 0.9 cm^2. He also had a dilated left atrial chamber. Ejection fraction was 52%. His basic metabolic panel was unremarkable, but he had an elevated pro-B-type natriuretic peptide level of 860 pg/dL and hemoglobin A1c level of 12%. The patient was started on cautious diuresis with furosemide to relieve congestion symptoms. He was referred for evaluation of aortic valve replacement.

Case Review

This patient had severe aortic stenosis and presented with symptoms of heart failure. He was optimized with medication therapy and considered for valve replacement surgery.

Case Discussion

Aortic stenosis develops from progressive calcification of leaflets with restriction of leaflet opening over time. Initially, the left ventricle compensates by increasing wall thickness (ie, hypertrophy). Later in the course, the left ventricle stiffens, and left ventricular diastolic pressure increases, contributing to dyspnea on exertion. In addition, the increased muscle mass results in decreased coronary flow reserve and angina. As noted, this patient had progressive degeneration of the aortic valve and presented with symptoms of heart failure.

Aortic stenosis develops from progressive calcification of leaflets with restriction of leaflet opening over time. Severe aortic stenosis is defined as an aortic valve area <1 cm^2 with a mean systolic Doppler gradient ≥40 mm Hg or a peak aortic velocity ≥4 m/s. For all symptomatic heart failure patients with classic symptoms such as angina, dyspnea, or syncope, valve replacement is indicated.

All patients presenting with acute decompensation should be optimized with medical therapy. In patients with aortic stenosis, diuretics and vasodilators should be used with caution. Depending on the valvular heart disease and patients' surgical risks, patients should be carefully selected for surgical treatment versus medical therapy.

Key Points

- Doppler echocardiography is indicated for evaluation of patients suspected of having aortic stenosis.
- Presence or absence of symptoms is crucial in management of aortic stenosis with heart failure.
- The risk of replacing valves must be weighed against the risk of delaying the procedure.
- Cardiology consults and co-management with the primary care physician are essential.

CASE 7

Heart Failure With Reduced Ejection Fraction and Device Therapy

A 70-year-old woman presented to the emergency department with shortness of breath, which occurred when performing everyday tasks such as bathing and walking a few steps. She slept in a recliner at night due to orthopnea. She had comorbidities of hypertension, dyslipidemia, and coronary artery disease (status post myocardial infarction [MI] and percutaneous coronary intervention [PCI] 2 month age, stenting of proximal left anterior descending artery, and status post coronary artery bypass graft 5 years ago). She was a current smoker, with no drug abuse history. Her current home medications included furosemide 80 mg twice daily, atorvastatin 80 mg once daily, lisinopril 20 mg once daily, spironolactone 25 mg once daily, metoprolol succinate 25 mg once daily, and aspirin 81 mg once daily. On clinical examination, she was in respiratory distress and using accessory muscles of respiration. Her blood pressure was 146/84 mm Hg, heart rate was 86 bpm, and oxygen saturation was 88% on room air. She had elevated jugular venous pressure and 1+ pitting lower extremity edema. There was no tenderness in the abdomen or hepatomegaly. Her ECG showed a QRS complex of 162 milliseconds and left bundle branch block (LBBB) morphology. An echocardiogram demonstrated systolic dysfunction, mild mitral regurgitation, a dilated left atrium, and an ejection fraction (EF) of 30%. Laboratory results showed elevated troponin (not trending up), a pro-B-type natriuretic peptide level of 4000 pg/mL, and an unremarkable basic metabolic panel. She was started on a furosemide drip with strict input/output monitoring, along with daily weight measurements and electrolyte monitoring. She was transitioned to oral furosemide as an inpatient and was discharged with an appointment at the cardiology clinic, where her medical therapy was optimized. After 3 months, she was reevaluated and was less symptomatic, with repeat EF of 32%. She was evaluated for an implantable cardioverter-defibrillator (ICD) and cardiac resynchronization therapy (CRT) placement. A CRT defibrillator (CRT-D) was implanted.

Case Review

In this case, the patient presented with signs and symptoms of heart failure, which was supported by laboratory values, and given her recent history of MI, she was diagnosed as having a ventricular myocardial infarct causing heart failure.

Case Discussion

All cases of heart failure should be classified using the New York Heart Association (NYHA) functional scale to plan the treatment strategy. Device therapies establish mechanical synchrony and thus improve EF. Sudden cardiac death occurs in almost half of patients with heart failure with reduced EF (HFrEF) due to the underlying risk for arrythmias. To prevent this, an ICD is recommended for all patients with NYHA class II and III symptoms, EF of <35% on guideline-directed medical therapy (GDMT), and a life expectancy of 1 year. After PCI, GDMT should be continued for 3 to 6 months and then ICD evaluation should be considered if the left ventricular EF (LVEF) is persistently reduced.

ICDs treat ventricular arrhythmia, and CRTs improve left ventricular systolic function by resynchronizing ventricular contractions. CRT-D is a device that combines CRT and an ICD. It helps in keeping the synchrony of ventricles. If there is dyssynchrony due to arrhythmia, then the device sends a shock to restore the rhythm. CRT is recommended in HFrEF patients with NYHA class III and IV, LVEF of <35%, and LBBB with QRS duration of 150 milliseconds. It consists of leads placed in the right atria, right ventricle, and coronary sinus to synchronize right and left ventricles. All devices are associated with infection, inappropriate firing, and valvular regurgitation.

Key Points

- The decision to implant a device should take into account patients' preferences and their quality of life, the LVEF, and the absence of other diseases that may affect life expectancy.
- An ICD is used as primary or secondary prevention, with the intent to increase survival.
- CRT is recommended for symptomatic HFrEF patients in sinus rhythm with QRS duration of 150 milliseconds, LBBB morphology, and LVEF of <35% on optimal medical therapy.

CASE 8

Diagnosis and Management of Heart Failure With Preserved Ejection Fraction

A 68-year-old obese man presented to the emergency department with weakness, fatigue, and progressively worsening dyspnea for the past 1 month, along with leg swelling and decreased urination. Recently, he was treated for a urinary tract infection. For the past 1 week, his exercise tolerance decreased to <1 city block from a baseline of 2 to 3 city blocks. Additionally, he was unable to do simple activities of daily living such as bathing and cooking. He indicated that he sits propped up because it makes breathing easier, but he denied any chest pain. The past medical history was significant for hypertension and dyslipidemia. Furthermore, he was a former smoker and cocaine abuser but stopped both habits 6 years ago. There was no known family history of coronary artery disease. His medications included aspirin 81 mg daily, atorvastatin 40 mg nightly, and hydrochlorothiazide 25 mg daily. He admitted to nonadherence to the medical regimen. Upon arrival, he was noted to be in mild respiratory distress, using accessory muscles of respiration, and was hypertensive, with a blood pressure of 168/88 mm Hg, and tachycardic, with a heart rate of 102 bpm. The physical examination was notable for increased jugular venous pulsations, displaced apical impulse, third heart sound, and grade 3/6 holosystolic murmur at the lower left parasternal border and apex. Bibasilar rales and hepatomegaly were present. Chest roentgenography showed pulmonary vascular congestion. The 12-lead ECG was suggestive of left ventricular hypertrophy with repolarization changes. The complete blood count, comprehensive metabolic panel, and thyroid function testing were all within normal limits. The pro-B-type natriuretic peptide (pro-BNP) level was elevated to 560 pg/dL. He was administered bolus intravenous furosemide, and repeat physical examination demonstrated decreased rales. Transthoracic echocardiography (TTE) showed mildly reduced left ventricular ejection fraction (LVEF) of 53%, concentric left ventricular hypertrophy, left atrial volume index of 36 mL/m^2, left ventricular mass index (LVMI) ≥119 g/m^2, mean E/e′ ratio ≥15, and mean e′-septal and lateral wall of 4 cm/s. He was continued on 40 mg of intravenous bolus furosemide daily. A selective coronary arteriogram showed angiographically normal coronary artery anatomy. Finally, a diagnosis of heart failure with preserved ejection fraction (HFpEF) was made. He was started on an angiotensin receptor blocker (ARB) for afterload reduction and hypertension control. He was educated about sodium and water restriction, weight reduction, and adherence to hypertension medications and was given a follow-up appointment in the cardiology clinic 1 week after hospital discharge. In the clinic, he was given a referral to physical therapy for endurance and resistance training to improve physical functioning, exercise capacity, and cardiac function.

Case Review

This patient presented with symptoms and signs of decompensated heart failure (HF). On further evaluation, he was found to have a LVEF >50% and TTE findings suggestive of HFpEF. The clinical signs and symptoms together with an elevated pro-BNP level and objective evidence based on TTE support the diagnosis of HFpEF. He was begun on diuretics to relieve his symptoms. An ARB was added for hypertension control and afterload reduction.

Case Discussion

HFpEF and HF with reduced ejection fraction (HFrEF) are considered entirely separate entities. HFpEF accounts for approximately one-half of HF hospitalizations. HFpEF occurs in the setting of inadequate ventricular filling and relaxation, leading to left ventricular stiffness, fibrosis, and hence diastolic dysfunction. The diagnosis of HFpEF may be clinically challenging, and it can be often misdiagnosed because it has common symptoms similar to other medical conditions. Guidelines recommend that in addition to symptoms of HF, presence of an elevated pro-BNP level, TTE findings suggestive of underlying heart disease such as left ventricular end-diastolic pressure >16 mm Hg, E/e' ratio >15, LVMI >122 g/m², and left atrial volume index >40 mL/m² should also be present.

Current recommendations regarding HFpEF treatment is to control the symptoms and medical comorbidities, such as hypertension, by using diuretics (either loop or thiazide) and to equilibrate the volume status. Care should be taken when using diuretics because this group of HF patients is volume sensitive and slight changes in volume status can lead to acute kidney injury.

Patients should be educated about a low-sodium diet because it plays a pivotal role in reducing HFpEF exacerbations.

Most patients with HFpEF are heart rate dependent to enhance left ventricular pumping. Although there is no suggestion about target heart rate in this cohort, one should still be cautious in using heart rate–controlling medications because abrupt changes in heart rate should be avoided.

The incidence of atrial fibrillation (AF) is seen more commonly in HFpEF patients, with similar characteristics, outcomes, and therapeutics as in HFrEF. Management of comorbid conditions is suggested to treat AF in this group.

The role of angiotensin receptor-neprilysin inhibitors is still under evaluation for the HFpEF population. Unlike for HFrEF, there is no therapy that has shown clear evidence of improvement in mortality in these patients. β-Adrenergic antagonists, certain ARBs, and mineralocorticoid receptor antagonist (MRA) therapies may be initiated. In fact, MRA therapy can prevent HF hospitalization in this group of patients.

Key Points

- HFpEF is a diagnostic challenge, and it is recommended to screen patients for both cardiovascular and noncardiovascular comorbidities, which if present should be treated.
- Based on current guidelines the following 4 criteria should be met to diagnose HFpEF: (1) presence of symptoms and/or signs of HF; (2) preserved LVEF ≥50% (or 40% to 49% for HF with midrange LVEF); (3) elevated levels of natriuretic peptides (BNP >35 pg/mL and/or N-terminal pro-BNP >125 pg/mL); and (4) objective evidence of other cardiac functional and structural alterations underlying HF.

CASE 9

Heart Failure With Preserved Ejection Fraction and Risk Factor Control

A 78-year-old morbidly obese woman was admitted to the telemetry floor with dyspnea during activities of daily living, such as walking to the bathroom and doing the laundry. She was unable to sleep at night due to orthopnea. This had progressively worsened over the past week and had been associated with wheezing and pinkish phlegm production at certain times. She felt fatigued constantly and reported intermittent palpitations. Additionally, she noticed swelling of both her legs up to the middle of the calf. The medical comorbidities included hypertension, dyslipidemia, and paroxysmal atrial fibrillation (PAF). She was a current chronic smoker (1.5 packs daily for 42 years). There was no drug abuse history. The current medical regimen included furosemide 40 mg twice daily, lisinopril 20 mg daily, metoprolol succinate 25 mg daily, and warfarin 3 mg nightly. The vital signs were as follows: blood pressure of 172/92 mm Hg, heart rate of 118 bpm (irregular), and saturation of 92% on room air. On physical examination, she was noted to be in respiratory distress using accessory muscles, and she had elevated jugular venous pulsations and 1+ pitting edema of the bilateral lower extremities. Furthermore, there was a third heart sound, hepatomegaly, and rales throughout both lung fields. The 12-lead ECG showed atrial fibrillation (AF) with left ventricular hypertrophy. Chest roentgenography revealed pulmonary vascular congestion. A transthoracic echocardiogram (TTE) demonstrated left ventricular ejection fraction (LVEF) of 54%, elevated E/e′ ratio >14, increased left atrial volume index >36 mL/m^2, and elevated noninvasive left ventricular filling pressure. The laboratory results showed a pro-B-type natriuretic peptide (pro-BNP) level of 560 pg/mL and unremarkable basic and comprehensive metabolic panels. She was started on a continuous intravenous furosemide infusion with strict input/output monitoring, along with daily weight measurements and electrolyte monitoring. The other medications were resumed. She had a net negative water balance. Repeat chest radiography showed no further congestion. She was offered invasive cardiac catheterization to look for coronary artery disease (CAD), which she refused. The medications were optimized on discharge, and she was given an appointment at the congestive heart failure clinic in 1 week. She went to the appointment and was advised to follow a heart healthy diet and an active lifestyle, to stop smoking, and to resume her previous home medications.

Case Review

This patient had multiple risk factors for heart failure with preserved ejection fraction (HFpEF). Based on clinical and imaging criteria, the patient was diagnosed with HFpEF and appropriately started on diuretic therapy. During the diastolic phase, the heart relaxes and fills with blood. In HFpEF, the left ventricle of the heart is unable to adequately fill with blood during diastole, thereby reducing the amount of blood pumped into the aorta. When the left ventricle becomes stiff or thickened, the pressure increases inside the left ventricle, and this causes blood to build up in left atrium, which causes pulmonary congestion of the lungs and, consequently, symptoms of heart failure (HF).

Case Discussion

Risk factors for HFpEF are older age, white race, diabetes mellitus, cigarette smoking, hypertension, obesity, CAD (other than myocardial infarction), anemia, and AF. Usually >1 comorbid condition is associated with HFpEF, but not with HF with reduced ejection fraction (HFrEF). With advancing age, the heart muscle stiffens, preventing the heart from filling with blood properly. Although HFpEF cannot be prevented, there are certain steps that can be taken to lower the risk. Treatment is largely empiric, and therapy focuses on avoiding tachycardia, treating congestion, maintaining normal atrial contraction when possible, and revascularization for CAD.

Patients should be counseled to quit smoking, increase activity as tolerated, maintain a healthy weight, and eat a heart-healthy diet, which involves limiting sugar and saturated fat and eating plenty of fruits, vegetables, whole grains, and low-fat dairy products. Smoking contributes to damage by stiffening the blood vessels, reducing the amount of oxygen in the blood, and making the heart beat faster.

Pharmacologic therapy includes use of diuretics to promote urination and reduce pulmonary congestion; β-adrenergic blockers to reduce blood pressure and tachycardia, thereby prolonging left ventricular diastolic filling time; and angiotensin-converting enzyme (ACE) inhibitors or angiotensin receptor blockers (ARBs) to improve blood flow by decreasing afterload. Mineralocorticoid receptor antagonists (MRAs) can be used to prevent HF hospitalization.

Surgical therapy would depend on the cause of HFpEF. Stress testing can be performed to determine if a patient has CAD, with subsequent cardiac catheterization if mandated. Surgery for repair of valves such as aortic or mitral valves based on guidelines can help in treating HFpEF.

Key Points

- HFpEF is a challenging diagnosis, so be thorough and consider invasive hemodynamic testing to confirm the diagnosis.
- Therapy focuses on avoiding tachycardia, treating congestion, and maintaining normal atrial contraction when possible.
- Although β-adrenergic blockers, ACE inhibitors, and ARBs have not shown a clear benefit in randomized clinical trials, they can be used to treat risk factors.
- MRAs do have a role in preventing HF hospitalization in this group of patients.

CASE 10

Heart Failure With Preserved Ejection Fraction and Arrhythmia Management

A 66-years old obese man was admitted to the telemetry floor with complaints of dyspnea that began about 3 weeks ago and was progressively worsening. His exercise tolerance decreased from 6 city blocks to 1 city block, and he had a 2-pillow orthopnea. He reported experiencing palpitations for the past week. This had never happened before, and there was no history of weight loss or cold intolerance. He denied chest pain, dizziness, and syncope. He did not drink caffeinated drinks or use any recreational drugs. His other medical comorbidities included diabetes mellitus, heart failure with preserved ejection fraction (HFpEF; left ventricular ejection fraction [LVEF], 55%), hypertension, and sleep-disordered breathing with obstructive sleep apnea syndrome. There was no family history of sudden cardiac death. He had been prescribed treatment with hydralazine 50 mg 3 times daily, furosemide 20 mg daily, and metformin 1000 mg daily but had not been adherent to medications since his prescription expired. On physical examination, he was noted to be in mild distress. The vital signs included tachycardia to 160 bpm with an irregular pulse and respiratory rate of 18 breaths/min. The jugular venous pulsations were measured to 8 cm H_2O. The patient had coarse bibasilar rales, a grade 2/3 holosystolic murmur at the apex radiating to the axilla, and bipedal edema. The 12-lead ECG showed rapid atrial fibrillation (AF) with a ventricular rate of 145 bpm. Highly sensitive cardiac troponin T levels were elevated but not trending upward. The pro-B-type natriuretic peptide level was 520 pg/dL. The comprehensive metabolic panel and thyroid function tests were within normal limits. Chest roentgenography showed pulmonary vascular congestion and mild cardiomegaly. He was administered metoprolol 5 mg by slow intravenous push, and the heart rate decreased to 90 bpm with continued AF. He was started on rivaroxaban, metoprolol succinate 25 mg daily, and enteral amiodarone 400 mg 2 times daily.

Case Review

In this case, the patient presented with an acute onset of dyspnea for 3 weeks. Furthermore, the physical examination was suggestive of heart failure (HF) with 12-lead ECG showing rapid AF. He was suspected of having an exacerbation of HFpEF secondary to arrhythmia. With adequate heart rate control, the patient's HF symptoms resolved. Restoration of normal sinus rhythm or control of ventricular rate suggests the tachycardia itself as underlying cause of myopathy.

Case Discussion

AF is the most common arrhythmia in HF, and the 2 conditions often coexist. In patients with known HF, new-onset AF is associated with worse prognosis, whereas incident HF precipitated by AF is more benign. Even the slightest change in heart rate can precipitate exacerbation. There is a complex interplay between AF and HF, with the mechanism still remaining poorly understood. AF causes structural and functional remodeling of the left atrium. AF causes left atrial dilation, impaired atrial function, atrial fibrosis, and left ventricular myocardial fibrosis, thus leading to diastolic dysfunction and atrioventricular annular remodeling with progressive mitral and tricuspid regurgitation. In permanent AF, chronic depletion of atrial natriuretic peptide may result in more vasoconstriction and congestion.

The basic principle of management includes controlling the arrhythmia causing HF, as evident in this case, and restoring normal sinus rhythm if possible. Identifying any precipitating factors and secondary causes of AF as well as possible correction plays an important role in the treatment. Volume management and risk factor control can help to avoid recurrence.

Key Points

- In HFpEF, symptoms of exacerbation can improve with adequate heart rate control.
- AF is associated with worse prognosis in HFpEF.

6

10 Real Cases on Hypertensive Emergency and Pericardial Disease: Diagnosis, Management, and Follow-Up

Niel Shah • Fareeha S. Alavi • Muhammad Saad

CASE 1

Management of Hypertensive Encephalopathy

A 45-year-old man with a 2-month history of progressive headache presented to the emergency department with nausea, vomiting, visual disturbance, and confusion for 1 day. He denied fever, weakness, numbness, shortness of breath, and flulike symptoms. He had significant medical history of hypertension and was on a β-blocker in the past, but a year ago, he stopped taking medication due to an unspecified reason. The patient denied any history of tobacco smoking, alcoholism, and recreational drug use. The patient had a significant family history of hypertension in both his father and mother. Physical examination was unremarkable, and at the time of triage, his blood pressure (BP) was noted as 195/123 mm Hg, equal in both arms. The patient was promptly started on intravenous labetalol with the goal to reduce BP by 15% to 20% in the first hour. The BP was rechecked after an hour of starting labetalol and was 165/100 mm Hg. MRI of the brain was performed in the emergency department and demonstrated multiple scattered areas of increased signal intensity on T2-weighted and fluid-attenuated inversion recovery (FLAIR) images in both the occipital and posterior parietal lobes. There were also similar lesions in both hemispheres of the cerebellum (especially the cerebellar white matter on the left) as well as in the medulla oblongata. The lesions were not associated with mass effect, and after contrast administration, there was no evidence of abnormal enhancement. In the emergency department, his BP decreased to 160/95 mm Hg, and he was transitioned from drip to oral medications and transferred to the telemetry floor. How would you manage this case?

Case Review

The patient initially presented with headache, nausea, vomiting, blurred vision, and confusion. The patient's BP was found to be 195/123 mm Hg, and MRI of the brain demonstrated scattered lesions with increased intensity in the occipital and posterior parietal lobes, as well as in cerebellum and medulla oblongata. The clinical presentation, elevated BP, and brain MRI findings were suggestive of hypertensive emergency, more specifically hypertensive encephalopathy. These MRI changes can be seen particularly in posterior reversible encephalopathy syndrome (PRES), a sequela of hypertensive encephalopathy. BP was initially controlled by labetalol, and after satisfactory control of BP, the patient was switched to oral antihypertensive medications.

Case Discussion

Hypertensive emergency refers to the elevation of systolic BP >180 mm Hg and/or diastolic BP >120 mm Hg that is associated with end-organ damage; however, in some conditions such as pregnancy, more modest BP elevation can constitute an emergency. An equal degree of hypertension but without end-organ damage constitutes a hypertensive urgency, the treatment of which requires gradual BP reduction over several hours. Patients with hypertensive emergency require rapid, tightly controlled reductions in BP that avoid overcorrection. Management typically occurs in an intensive care setting with continuous arterial BP monitoring and continuous infusion of antihypertensive agents.

Clinical Symptoms

An expedited evaluation for the cause of hypertension as well as assessment for the presence of end-organ failure, including encephalopathy, focal neurologic deficits (including vision changes), myocardial ischemia, heart failure, and acute kidney injury, should be performed. Diagnostic studies should be driven by clinical suspicion.

Management

Optimal therapy, including the choice of agent and the BP goal, varies according to the specific hypertensive emergency. It is generally unwise to lower the BP too quickly or too much because ischemic damage can occur in vascular beds that have become habituated with the higher level of BP (ie, autoregulation). For most hypertensive emergencies, mean arterial pressure should be reduced gradually by approximately 10% to 20% in the first hour and by a further 5% to 15% over the next 23 hours. This often results in a target BP of <180/<120 mm Hg for the first hour and <160/<110 mm Hg for the next 23 hours (but rarely <130/<80 mm Hg during that time frame).

The major exceptions to gradual BP lowering over the first day are as follows:

- The acute phase of an ischemic stroke: The BP is usually not lowered unless it is ≥185/110 mm Hg in patients who are candidates for reperfusion therapy or ≥220/120 mm Hg in patients who are not candidates for reperfusion (thrombolytic) therapy.
- Acute aortic dissection: The systolic BP should be rapidly lowered to a target of 100 to 120 mm Hg (to be attained in 20 minutes) to reduce aortic shearing forces.
- Intracerebral hemorrhage: Goals of antihypertensive therapy in such patients are variable and are discussed elsewhere.

After a suitable period (often 8 to 24 hours) of BP control at target in the intensive care unit, oral medications are usually given, and the initial intravenous therapy is tapered and discontinued.

Key Points

- Hypertensive encephalopathy or PRES presents with nausea, vomiting, blurry vision, and headache.
- MRI features of scattered changes in the occipital area are characteristic of PRES.
- Gradual control of BP is the cornerstone of management.

CASE 2

Management of Renovascular Hypertension

A 55-year-old man was brought to the emergency department after he developed sudden onset of shortness of breath for 1 day associated with difficulty in sleeping and even speaking full sentences. He had 2 prior hospitalizations with the same complaint during which he was noted to have a hypertensive emergency that was treated with antihypertensive medications. He denied fever, flulike symptoms, chest pain, and vomiting. His medications included lisinopril, amlodipine, and furosemide. He stated that he is adherent on medications. He had a significant medical history of poorly controlled chronic hypertension. He did not know his family history. Social history was significant for current cigarette smoking of 1 pack per day for the past 30 years. In the emergency department, the initial blood pressure reading was 230/150 mm Hg with room air oxygen saturation of 92%. The patient was found to be in mild distress. Complete physical examination showed bilateral rales in all lung fields with audible S_4 heart sound. The rest of the physical examination was unremarkable. ECG showed left ventricular hypertrophy, and chest x-ray showed diffuse interstitial pattern infiltrates suggestive of pulmonary edema. Laboratory data showed elevated creatinine, troponin, and pro-B-type natriuretic peptide (pro-BNP). He was started on nasal oxygen inhalation, and 1 intravenous dose of furosemide was administered. He started feeling significant improvement, and the BP decreased to 170/110 mm Hg. He was transferred to the telemetry floor for further management. How would you manage this case?

Case Review

This patient presented with flash pulmonary edema in the setting of hypertensive emergency. The typical presentation, the examination findings, and improvement with diuretic are characteristic for renovascular hypertension. Another important aspect in this case is the recurrent hospitalizations with similar complaints, especially after initiation of an angiotensin-converting enzyme inhibitor (ACEI), and this patient should be evaluated for renal artery stenosis. Elevated troponin and pro-BNP are suggestive of fluid overload status.

Case Discussion

Kidney disease can be a complication of hypertension, which can lead to organ damage. The presence of renovascular disease cannot predict renovascular hypertension (ie, renal artery stenosis). Renovascular hypertension is identified by acute kidney injury as a result of renal hypoperfusion, leading to a renin-angiotensin surge that ultimately causes vasoconstriction and hypertension. Renin/aldosterone levels will be high in renal artery stenosis, but with bilateral involvement, they can be normal or low, causing volume-dependent hypertension. The most common cause of renal artery stenosis is atherosclerosis. Fibromuscular dysplasia is a rare cause and usually suspected in young woman.

Clinical Symptoms

Recurrent flash pulmonary edema with creatinine elevation even with controlled blood pressure is the most common presenting feature. The symptoms can be worsened by the recent initiation of an ACEI. Renal bruit is an insensitive examination finding that can be observed in a few cases.

Management

Duplex ultrasound can be an initial screening test, with the gold standard diagnostic tests being CT or magnetic resonance angiography. Use of contrast is generally avoided unless surgical intervention is planned. Renin/aldosterone levels do not aid in diagnosis.

Treatment strategy includes aggressive cardiovascular risk factor modification. Percutaneous intervention with angioplasty and stenting can be considered in select patients with recurrent flash pulmonary edema, bilateral renal artery stenosis, or fibromuscular dysplasia. The clinical studies have not shown any benefit of intervention over medical therapy. Blood pressure control should be optimized in these patients.

Key Points

- Recurrent flash pulmonary edema is the initial presentation of renovascular hypertension, along with creatinine elevation especially after initiation of ACEI.
- Duplex ultrasound is the initial screening test for the diagnosis.
- Treatment includes management of blood pressure and other cardiovascular risk factors.

CASE 3

Management of Sympathomimetic Drug Overdose

A 52-year-old woman was brought to the emergency department after being found walking in the middle of a freeway on a ramp. She was given intramuscular haloperidol by emergency medical personnel for agitation on the way to the hospital. Her medical history was notable for polysubstance use. On physical examination in the emergency department, she was alert and restless. Vitals were noted as temperature of 38.2°C (100.8°F), blood pressure of 210/124 mm Hg, pulse rate of 124 bpm, respiration rate of 14 breaths/min, and oxygen saturation of 97% breathing ambient air. Her pupils were symmetric, dilated, and reactive to light. Slight tremor of the hands was noted. No tongue fasciculations were observed. The skin was warm and diaphoretic. The chest was clear to auscultation. The patient was given intravenous benzodiazepines and started on fluids, and cultures were sent. Laboratory studies revealed a serum creatine kinase level of 6600 U/L, an increase in creatinine level from a baseline of 0.9 mg/dL to 1.4 mg/dL, and a normal troponin level. Urinary toxicology was positive for cocaine. Fractional excretion of sodium was <1%. An ECG revealed sinus tachycardia without ischemic changes. After initial control of blood pressure with diltiazem, the patient was admitted to the telemetry floor for further workup and management. How would you manage this case?

Case Review

In this case, the combination of hypertension, tachycardia, fever, diaphoresis, mydriasis, and rhabdomyolysis is most consistent with sympathomimetic intoxication. Common causes of sympathomimetic intoxication include cocaine, amphetamines, ephedrine, and caffeine. In this patient, recent use of cocaine was suspected to be the reason behind the patient's presentation because urine toxicology was positive for cocaine. Clinical presentation, history of cocaine use, physical examination findings, and urine toxicology results were suggestive of sympathomimetic intoxication caused by cocaine use. The patient was treated with gentle hydration, benzodiazepines, and antihypertensive medications.

Case Discussion

Sympathomimetic toxicity is commonly seen in the United States, either due to overdose of over-the-counter medications (ephedrine-based cough syrup) or street drugs such as cocaine and methylamphetamines. These drugs exert psychological and physiologic toxic effects, leading to central nervous system stimulation and organ damage. The toxic effects commonly encountered on a medical floor are psychosis, seizure, acute kidney injury, coronary vasospasm, rhabdomyolysis, hypoglycemia, and hypertensive crisis.

Clinical Symptoms

Symptoms include tachycardia, hypertension, diaphoresis, seizure, hyperthermia, nausea, vomiting, agitation, and combativeness.

Management

The diagnostic process includes a routine laboratory test to check thyroid function, ECG, measurement of creatine kinase levels and electrolytes, and kidney function test. Imaging of the head can be done based on neurologic findings. Urine drug screen should be performed; however, some of the newer drugs cannot be detected on routine toxicology screening. Blood cultures and other septic workup can be obtained to exclude other etiologies of fever.

Treatment strategy consists of benzodiazepines as first-line therapy for sympathomimetic intoxication. Experience in patients with cocaine-induced hypertension suggests use of β-blockers can paradoxically worsen hypertension due to loss of β-mediated vascular smooth muscle relaxation. Given these concerns with cocaine, it is reasonable to avoid β-blockers, such as propranolol, in sympathomimetic intoxication in general. Furthermore, acute kidney injury can be due to a combination of hypertensive renal crisis or dehydration and rhabdomyolysis, which would mandate hydration and rapid, tightly controlled blood pressure reduction. Another aspect of management is monitoring for arrythmia on telemetry to prevent any cardiac event in 24 to 48 hours. Patient should also be monitored for seizures.

Key Points

- Sympathomimetic toxicity is commonly observed in the United States, with presenting symptoms including agitation, bizarre behavior, tremors, hypertension, and seizures.
- Routine assessment of thyroid function, creatine kinase, kidney function, and electrolytes should be performed.
- Benzodiazepine as the first-line treatment, control of blood pressure, and prevention of organ damage are the cornerstones of management.

CASE 4

Management of Resistant Hypertension

A 55-year-old African American man was sent to the emergency department from the primary care physician's clinic for markedly elevated blood pressure not controlled with clinic medications. He went to the clinic for follow-up of uncontrolled blood pressure. The blood pressure in the clinic was noted as 190/120 mm Hg and was equal in both arms. He stated that he took his medications in the morning. This was his third clinic visit with uncontrolled blood pressure. He remained asymptomatic otherwise. His only medical history was hypertension. His medications included amlodipine 10 mg, lisinopril 20 mg, and hydrochlorothiazide 25 mg. He reported no smoking, no over-the-counter medication use, and no substance abuse. Family history was significant for a brother with diabetes. He denied chest pain, shortness of breath, abdominal complaints, and urinary complaints. Physical examination was significant for severe hypertension with blood pressure of 215/125 mm Hg and heart rate of 75 bpm. Body mass index (BMI) was noted as 27 kg/m^2. Otherwise, his examination was unremarkable. Initial laboratory data showed creatinine of 1.5 mg/dL (baseline 1.2 mg/dL); otherwise, no lab abnormalities of acute significance were noted. He was given 1 dose of intravenous labetalol in the emergency department, and the blood pressure came down to 160/95 mm Hg. He was transferred to the telemetry floor for further evaluation. How would you manage this case?

Case Review

This case described the management of resistant hypertension. Poorly controlled blood pressure despite use of 3 medications should be evaluated for resistant hypertension. Although the patient was adherent to his medications, the blood pressure was still uncontrolled. First, measures should be taken to exclude pseudo-resistance by assuring proper technique, detailed review of the medication list and over-the-counter medications use, and assessing for white coat hypertension and lifestyle-related causes. In this case, the blood pressure was controlled with home medications in the hospital. In addition, the patient had recently started using nonsteroidal anti-inflammatory drugs, for the headache, which could a cause of his poorly controlled blood pressure.

Case Discussion

Resistant hypertension is defined as blood pressure above goal despite use of 3 antihypertensive medications. Diuretics should be the part of the medication regimen before labeling hypertension as resistant. The incidence varies from 5% to 10% and is more common in older patients, African Americans, and obese patients. Pseudo-resistance should be excluded before making the diagnosis, after which an identifiable cause should be investigated. Resistant hypertension is undoubtedly associated with increased cardiovascular risk.

Clinical Symptoms

Symptoms of uncontrolled blood pressure include nausea, vomiting, headache, chest pain, shortness of breath, and vision changes. A majority of the cases remain asymptomatic.

Management

Management of resistant hypertension starts with thorough history and physical examination to identify causes of hypertension that will suggest appropriate testing. Alcohol intake screening should be performed along with evaluation for sleep apnea. Thyroid function tests, kidney function tests, parathyroid/calcium levels, renin-aldosterone-cortisol pathway assessment, and necessary imaging for renal vascular hypertension and aortic disease can be performed.

The ideal antihypertensive regimen for resistant hypertension includes diuretics, calcium channel blockers, and renin-aldosterone system agents. Aldosterone antagonist can be added in addition to optimize blood pressure control. Administration of one long-acting medication at night time can help in achieving blood pressure targets early. Appropriate lifestyle changes and adherence to medications should be reinforced.

Key Points

- Resistant hypertension consists of blood pressure not reaching goal despite 3 antihypertensive medications, 1 of which is a diuretic.
- Management involves identifying the cause of uncontrolled hypertension by clinical correlation. Optimization of antihypertensive medications is the cornerstone of management.

CASE 5

Management of Hypertension in a Hemodialysis Patient

A 65-year-old man presented to the emergency department (ED) with a complaint of shortness of breath for 1 day. He received his regular dialysis session 2 days prior but started feeling the symptoms 1 day after dialysis. He denied chest pain, fever, headache, dizziness, and weakness. He had multiple hospitalizations for uncontrolled blood pressure despite adherence on medications and to dialysis sessions. He was referred to a nutritionist and, since then, followed a strict low-sodium diet. His medical history included hypertension, coronary artery disease, diabetes mellitus, and hyperlipidemia. He had been receiving hemodialysis for the past 4 years through a left arm arteriovenous graft 3 times a week. He denied any significant social history or family history. Medications included losartan, nifedipine extended release, labetalol, aspirin, and atorvastatin. On presentation to the ED, the vital signs were noted as blood pressure of 220/125 mm Hg, equal in both arms; oxygen saturation of 98% on room air; pulse of 80 bpm; and respiratory rate 16 breaths/min. Physical examination was significant for mild distress and rales in all lung fields. The rest of the examination was insignificant. His ECG showed left ventricular hypertrophy, and the chest x-ray showed diffuse infiltrates suggestive of pulmonary edema. Electrolytes were normal except creatinine of 7.5 mg/dL. The renal team was consulted, and he received a hemodialysis session in the ED, after which he started feeling better and the blood pressure trended down to 160/90 mm Hg. He was transferred to the telemetry floor for further management. How would you manage this case?

Case Review

This case describes the management of hypertension in end-stage renal disease. Medication management and optimization of the dialysis session are key to treatment in this case.

Case Discussion

The majority of patients on hemodialysis are hypertensive. Excessive activation of the renin-angiotensin-aldosterone system and sympathetic system causes difficulty in maintaining optimal blood pressure in these patients. Elevated systolic blood pressure is associated with increased mortality in these patients. The causes of poorly controlled blood pressure in this population include underestimation of dry weight, nonadherence to salt and water intake, low doses of antihypertensive medications and their nonoptimization over 24 hours, and the practice of discontinuing therapy before dialysis. Paradoxical hypertension is observed at the end of the dialysis session, which is precipitated by hypovolemia, hypercalcemia, high hematocrit level, and improved oxygenation.

Management

Optimization of the dialysis session includes free water and salt restriction. A longer duration of sessions with low ultrafiltration rate, hemodialysis at night, and short daily sessions can be used to reduce dialysate sodium content and have shown benefit in blood pressure improvement.

Optimization of antihypertensive medications includes use of combinations such as angiotensin receptor blockers/angiotensin-converting enzyme inhibitors along with calcium channel blockers. Calcium channel blockers have a unique role in dialysis patients with volume expansion, and its pharmacokinetics remain unaltered in end-stage renal disease patients. β-Blockers can be used as an adjunct to this regimen. Second-line treatment includes clonidine and minoxidil. Paradoxical hypertension can be treated using nifedipine or captopril and by identifying the causative factor. There is no target blood pressure range for dialysis patients, but consensus is to keep it <140/90 mm Hg and <130/80 mm Hg before and after dialysis, respectively.

Key Points

- Management of hypertension in dialysis patients consists of identification of the cause.
- Medication management and optimization of dialysis session should be emphasized.

CASE 6

Management of Effusive Constrictive Pericarditis

A 47-year-old man presented to the emergency department with a 6-week history of progressive fatigue, dyspnea on exertion, and vague chest "fullness." He also had pedal edema for the past 2 weeks. His past medical history was unknown. He had no history of incarceration or recent travel and was not immunocompromised. No significant family history was found. On physical examination, temperature was 37.5°C (99.5°F), blood pressure was 132/76 mm Hg with pulsus paradoxus of 16 mm Hg, pulse rate was 100 bpm, and respiration rate was 16 breaths/min. The jugular veins were distended to the angle of the mandible. The lungs were clear to auscultation. No diastolic sound or pericardial friction rub was noted. Hepatomegaly was present. Pitting edema was noted bilaterally at the ankles. Laboratory studies showed erythrocyte sedimentation rate of 86 mm/h and leukocyte count of 11,000/μL (11×10^9/L) with normal differential. An ECG showed sinus tachycardia with a nonspecific ST-T–wave abnormality. A chest radiograph revealed an enlarged cardiac silhouette without pericardial calcification. The patient was admitted to the telemetry floor for further workup and management. How would you manage this case?

Case Review

This patient had subacute signs of elevated right heart pressure. Pulsus paradoxus was present on examination. Echocardiogram should be performed for pericardial effusion, and if fluid is present, it should be drained and studied. He should be tested for HIV, connective tissue disease, and tuberculosis. In this case, echocardiogram demonstrated a moderately sized pericardial effusion with evidence of tamponade. The intrapericardial pressure remained elevated and equalized despite drainage, consistent with a diagnosis of effusive constrictive pericarditis.

Case Discussion

Effusive constrictive pericarditis is caused by obstruction of the pericardial space by visceral pericardium. It is characterized by the persistence of elevated right atrial pressure after intrapericardial pressure has been reduced to normal levels by removal of pericardial fluid. Effusive constrictive pericarditis may occur following idiopathic or infectious pericarditis or radiation therapy. CT or cardiac MRI may demonstrate thickening of the pericardium, but calcification is usually absent.

Clinical Symptoms

Symptoms include chest pain, shortness of breath, fatigue, and pedal edema. Symptoms can start at any time after acute pericarditis, ranging from 3 to 26 months.

Management

Nonsteroidal anti-inflammatory drugs and colchicine are first-line therapy, similar to acute pericarditis. Close follow-up is recommended. Pericardiectomy may be required in patients with pericarditis that does not respond to pharmacologic therapy. Extensive epicardiectomy is required in such refractory cases. In a few cases of tamponade, effusive pericarditis can be missed. Idiopathic cases are usually self-resolving, and no dedicated diagnosis or treatment is required.

Key Points

- Effusive constrictive pericarditis can be seen after radiation therapy and infections. The majority of cases remain idiopathic.
- Idiopathic cases are self-resolving. The other cases can be managed using conservative therapy. Surgery is an option for refractory cases.

CASE 7

Management of Cardiac Tamponade

A 55-year-old man presented to the emergency department for a 1-day history of worsening dyspnea and a 1-month history of increasing weight and peripheral edema. He had a long-standing history of poorly controlled hypertension and stage IV chronic kidney disease. Minoxidil and hydralazine were added to his medical regimen 2 months ago. His other medications included labetalol, a clonidine patch, and furosemide. No significant family or social history was noted. On physical examination, he was in distress, with increased work of breathing and diaphoresis. Temperature was normal, blood pressure was 90/60 mm Hg with pulsus paradoxus of 18 mm Hg, pulse rate was 118 bpm, and respiration rate was 25 breaths/min. Oxygen saturation was 90% on breathing ambient air. Jugular venous distention was present. Heart sounds were distant, and no pericardial friction rub or murmur was noted. Crackles were noted at the lower quarter of both lung fields. Pitting edema was present up to the level of the knees. Laboratory studies revealed a blood urea nitrogen level of 86 mg/dL, a serum creatinine level of 5.1 mg/dL, and a serum potassium level of 5.0 mEq/L (5.0 mmol/L). A chest radiograph showed an enlarged cardiac silhouette, prominent pulmonary vasculature, and evidence of pulmonary edema. ECG was noted to have low voltage. The patient was admitted to the telemetry floor for further management. How would you manage this case?

Case Review

This case represents typical signs of cardiac tamponade, which include tachycardia, hypotension, muffled heart sounds, elevation of the jugular venous pulse, and pulsus paradoxus. ECG in cardiac tamponade may show electrical alternans or low voltage. This patient was taking minoxidil and hydralazine, both of which may be associated with the development of a pericardial effusion. He was started on intravenous fluids. Echocardiographic findings were compatible with cardiac tamponade. The patient underwent pericardiocentesis and tolerated the procedure well.

Case Discussion

Cardiac tamponade occurs when fluid accumulation within the pericardial space compresses the heart and impedes diastolic filling. When fluid accumulates rapidly (such as with trauma, aortic dissection, or invasive cardiac procedures), tamponade may occur at relatively low pericardial volumes. Subacute or chronic processes, such as neoplastic disease or hypothyroidism, may be associated with much larger effusions (several hundred milliliters in volume).

Clinical Symptoms

Clinical signs of tamponade include tachycardia, hypotension, muffled heart sounds, and elevation of the jugular venous pulse. The y descent of the jugular venous pulse may be absent because passive filling of the ventricles is impeded by the intrapericardial pressure. This finding may be difficult to appreciate, especially in a patient with tachycardia. Pulsus paradoxus represents exaggerated ventricular interdependence and is a key clinical feature of cardiac tamponade. It is characterized by a fall in systolic pressure of >10 mm Hg during inspiration. Pulsus paradoxus is not specific for tamponade and must be interpreted in conjunction with other clinical and echocardiographic features.

Diagnostic Evaluation

The ECG may demonstrate electrical alternans (related to a swinging motion of the heart within the pericardial fluid) or low voltage in patients with tamponade. If the accumulation of fluid has occurred slowly, the cardiac silhouette is typically enlarged on chest radiography.

Echocardiography is an essential tool in the diagnosis of cardiac tamponade because it defines the presence, distribution, and relative volume of pericardial fluid. Early diastolic collapse of the right ventricle, late diastolic collapse of the right atrium, and abnormal inter-ventricular septal motion are features associated with cardiac tamponade. Additionally, Doppler evaluation may demonstrate a decrease in mitral inflow velocity of >25% with inspiration, which is the echocardiographic equivalent of pulsus paradoxus.

Cardiac catheterization is rarely necessary for the diagnosis. The hemodynamic hall-marks of tamponade include blunting or loss of the y descent within the right atrial pressure waveform and elevated and equalized diastolic pressures. The latter reflects the transmitted effect of the intrapericardial pressure. Invasive arterial pressure recordings also show pulsus paradoxus.

Management

Cardiac tamponade is life threatening, and once a diagnosis is established, fluid removal is required. Drainage is most commonly accomplished with pericardiocentesis, with flu-oroscopy or echocardiographic guidance. Surgical therapy via a subxiphoid approach is indicated to drain fluid when pericardiocentesis cannot be performed safely, to obtain pericardial tissue for diagnostic purposes, or to prevent recurrent pericardial effusion by creating a pericardial window (often used in cases of malignant pericardial effusion). In hemodynamically unstable patients, intravenous normal saline is used to stabilize the patient as a temporizing measure or as a bridge to definitive therapy.

After drainage of pericardial fluid, hemodynamic and clinical evaluation may occa-sionally disclose findings of underlying pericardial constriction, termed *effusive constric-tive pericarditis*. If clinical evaluation and imaging techniques (eg, cardiac MRI) suggest an active inflammatory process, a course of medical therapy similar to that for acute pericardi-tis may be considered, and the patient should be reevaluated before surgery is contemplated.

Key Points

- Clinical signs of cardiac tamponade include tachycardia, hypotension, muffled heart sounds, elevation of the jugular venous pulse, and pulsus paradoxus.
- Patients with cardiac tamponade require drainage of pericardial fluid with pericardio-centesis. Surgical drainage is indicated when pericardiocentesis cannot be performed safely, pericardial tissue is needed for diagnostic purposes, or a pericardial window is required to prevent recurrent pericardial effusion

CASE 8

Management of Constrictive Pericarditis

A 68-year-old man presented to the emergency department for worsening lower extremity swelling. He had a 1-year history of bilateral lower extremity edema and abdominal dis-tention. Eight years ago, he had esophageal carcinoma treated with radiotherapy. Medical history was otherwise significant for hypertension, type 2 diabetes mellitus, and hyper-cholesterolemia. Medications were bumetanide, atorvastatin, metformin, and lisinopril. He used to smoke cigarettes, with a 20-pack-year history, but quit 5 years ago, and he denied any recreational drugs use or alcohol use. Family history was insignificant. On physical examination, the patient was afebrile, blood pressure was 174/90 mm Hg, pulse rate was 89 bpm, and respiration rate was normal. Jugular venous distention was present to the angle of the mandible while seated, with prominent pulsations. Cardiac examination revealed an early diastolic sound at the apex. The liver was palpable 5 cm below the costal margin. The abdomen was distended with ascites. There was bilateral pitting edema to the level of the thighs. Pulmonary examination revealed no crackles. Laboratory studies were significant for a B-type natriuretic peptide level of 96 pg/mL. Chest radiographs revealed pericardial calcification. A 12-lead ECG demonstrated normal sinus rhythm with normal QRS voltage. The patient was admitted to the telemetry floor for further workup and management. How would you manage this case?

Case Review

Patients with constrictive pericarditis most commonly present with indolent progression of right-sided heart failure symptoms, including peripheral edema, ascites, and fatigue. In this patient, signs of venous congestion predominate, pericardial calcification is present on the chest radiograph, and the serum B-type natriuretic peptide level is low, which suggest wall tension is not elevated. His echocardiogram demonstrated normal right and left ventricular size and function. Left ventricular wall thickness was normal. Mild tricuspid regurgitation was present. There was respiratory variation in the filling of the right and left ventricles, ventricular septal shift during respiration, and dilation of the inferior vena cava. The estimated right ventricular systolic pressure was 46 mm Hg. There was no pericardial effusion. He was started on diuretics and scheduled for pericardiectomy. He underwent pericardiectomy via median sternotomy.

Case Discussion

Constrictive pericarditis is characterized by pericardial thickening, fibrosis, and sometimes calcification that impair diastolic filling and limit total cardiac volume. In developed countries, most cases are viral or idiopathic in origin. Other causes include cardiac surgery, chest irradiation, autoimmune disease, and tuberculosis or other bacterial infection. Tuberculosis remains a major cause of constrictive pericarditis in developing countries.

Clinical Symptoms

Patients with constrictive pericarditis most commonly present with indolent progression of right-sided heart failure symptoms, including peripheral edema, abdominal swelling, and fatigue. Dyspnea and fatigue occur due to the increased diastolic pressures and limited ability to augment cardiac output due to the fixed stroke volume.

On physical examination, the jugular veins can be distended, with prominent x and y descents. The height of the waveform does not fall or may increase during inspiration (Kussmaul sign), reflecting the fixed diastolic volume of the right heart. Early diastolic filling is unimpaired or even accentuated and is followed by sudden cessation when total acceptable volume is met, resulting in a high-frequency early diastolic sound (the pericardial knock). Pulsus paradoxus is less frequent in constrictive pericarditis than in cardiac tamponade. Peripheral edema, ascites, hepatomegaly, and pleural effusions are common. Muscle wasting may be evident in advanced cases.

Diagnostic Evaluation

Constrictive pericarditis is diagnosed with imaging studies and hemodynamic evaluation. Chest radiography or CT may demonstrate partial or circumferential pericardial calcification, and CT or cardiac MRI may demonstrate pericardial thickening (>3 mm). Importantly, constriction may exist in the absence of these findings. In 1 case series, 18% of cases of hemodynamically proven constrictive pericarditis occurred with normal pericardial thickness. Cardiac MRI may also demonstrate an inspiratory septal shift, a sign of ventricular interdependence.

Transthoracic echocardiography in constrictive pericarditis represents normal right and left ventricular size and systolic function despite prominent symptoms and examination findings suggestive of heart failure. The echocardiographic finding of dilatation of the inferior vena cava reflects elevated right-sided filling (right atrial) pressure. Myocardial relaxation is impaired in myocardial disease, such as restrictive cardiomyopathy, but is unimpaired or even enhanced in constriction, in which early diastolic filling is rapid and unimpeded. Doppler echocardiography and tissue Doppler velocity are required to differentiate constrictive pericarditis from restrictive cardiomyopathy.

When constrictive pericarditis is suspected but not confirmed by echocardiography, cardiac catheterization can be performed. Invasive hemodynamic findings of constrictive pericarditis include a prominent y descent in the right atrial waveform, which corresponds with the dip of the right ventricular dip-and-plateau waveform (square root sign). The significant y descent and the right ventricular dip both represent unimpeded or rapid early diastolic ventricular filling. As inflow volume reaches the fixed pericardial constraint, pressure rises rapidly until maximum volume is achieved; pressure then remains constant, causing the plateau phase of the square root sign. A more specific finding is ventricular interdependence during simultaneous right and left ventricular systolic pressure measurement. During inspiration, right ventricular inflow is enhanced, and right ventricular systolic pressure rises; however, these changes occur with a concomitant decrease in left ventricular filling and reduction in left ventricular stroke volume and systolic pressure. The converse is seen during expiration.

Increased pericardial thickening and impaired distensibility may occur without fibrosis or calcification in the setting of acute or subacute inflammation. In these patients, constriction may be transient and resolve spontaneously. Patients with transient constrictive pericarditis present most commonly with symptoms of right-sided heart failure, although fever and chest pain may indicate the active inflammatory condition. Most cases are idiopathic; other causes include recent cardiac surgery, acute pericarditis, autoimmune disease, or chemotherapy. Systemic markers of inflammation (erythrocyte sedimentation rate and C-reactive protein) may be elevated in patients with transient constriction but are generally normal in patients with fixed constriction. Echocardiographic features are similar to those of fixed constriction; however, pericardial effusion is more likely to be present in patients with transient constrictive pericarditis.

Management

Treatment of transient constrictive pericarditis is the same as for acute pericarditis. Treatment with anti-inflammatory agents for 2 to 3 months is reasonable in hemodynamically stable patients before recommending surgical pericardiectomy. Response to therapy is monitored clinically and by echocardiographic features in combination with serologic markers.

Patients with chronic pericardial constriction should be referred for surgical pericardial stripping (pericardiectomy performed via median sternotomy). In advanced cases, adequate resection of the pericardium may be difficult, leading to incomplete resolution of symptoms. Diuretic therapy to relieve symptoms of congestion may be useful in patients who are not deemed surgical candidates or in whom stripping was incomplete.

Key Points

- Constrictive pericarditis is characterized by pericardial thickening, fibrosis, and sometimes calcification that impair diastolic filling and limit total cardiac volume.
- Transthoracic echocardiography is the initial diagnostic test for evaluating constrictive pericarditis; however, additional imaging may be required to differentiate constrictive pericarditis from restrictive cardiomyopathy.
- Patients with chronic pericardial constriction should be referred for surgical pericardial stripping (pericardiectomy performed via median sternotomy).

CASE 9

Management of Acute Myocarditis

A 45-year-old woman presented to the emergency department with complaints of worsening shortness of breath for the past week. The patient reported dyspnea on exertion after walking only 2 blocks, when walking upstairs, and sometimes at rest. Additionally, the patient was experiencing orthopnea and paroxysmal nocturnal dyspnea. She recalled a viral illness 2 weeks ago, during which she had a runny nose and body aches. She took herbal tea for a few days, and the symptoms resolved. The patient denied any palpitation, fever, recent travel, sick contacts, or joint pains. Review of systems was otherwise unremarkable. The patient had no past medical history, and past surgical history was significant for appendectomy. She denied use of tobacco, alcohol, or recreational drugs. She was living with her 2 kids and worked for a software company. No significant family history was reported. She was only taking cetirizine and multivitamins at home. On arrival, her vital signs were stable, with a blood pressure of 127/70 mm Hg, pulse of 83 bpm, respiratory rate of 17 breaths/min, temperature of 37.1°C (98.8°F), and oxygen saturation of 96% on room air. Physical examination was otherwise unremarkable except she appeared lethargic. Cardiovascular and lung examinations were unremarkable. Laboratory results showed significantly elevated troponin and pro-B-type natriuretic peptide. ECG showed nonspecific ST/T–wave changes. Chest radiograph showed enlarged heart shadow. The patient was admitted to the telemetry floor for further workup. How would you manage this case?

Case Review

This case describes a young woman with no comorbid conditions who presented with exertional dyspnea and heart failure symptoms. Recent viral illness was noted, and cardiac biomarkers were elevated. Although acute coronary syndrome is a consideration, based on the clinical data, sequence of events, and low-risk group, myocarditis seems to be the likely diagnosis. Echocardiogram should be performed to assess functioning of ventricles and to exclude any valvular or wall motion abnormalities. Malignant arrythmias should be monitored. Myocarditis is treated using conservative measures.

Case Discussion

Acute myocarditis presents as an acute heart failure syndrome that develops within days to weeks of an inciting event. It is usually preceded by viral illness, although the pathogenesis remains unclear. Various etiologies, including infectious or inflammatory causes, may be responsible, although a vast majority of cases remain idiopathic. The most common viral infections include adenovirus, coxsackievirus, and enterovirus.

Clinical Symptoms

A viral prodrome including fever, myalgias, and respiratory symptoms may be present. Heart failure symptoms include dyspnea, fatigue, chest pain, and arrythmias.

Management

Myocarditis is diagnosed by detailed history and physical examination. ECG may show subtle abnormalities with nonspecific ST/T–wave changes. Troponin levels are markedly elevated. Endomyocardial biopsy is indicated in the setting of ventricular arrythmias, high-grade conduction abnormalities, or lack of response to heart failure therapy. Biopsy in myocarditis shows myocardial necrosis and/or degeneration with surrounding inflammation.

Treatment consists of supportive measures and heart failure therapy. Immunosuppressants have not shown any benefit in mortality and improvement of ejection fraction. Recovery time is usually 6 to 12 months. Because half of cases recover by 1 year, an implantable cardioverter-defibrillator should not be placed until after 6 months of heart failure therapy.

Giant cell myocarditis is a fulminant form of myocarditis manifested, in the younger population, by ventricular arrythmias and cardiac dysfunction despite medical therapy. Immunosuppressant therapy has shown survival benefit in this entity with role for cardiac transplantation and ventricular assist devices.

Key Points

- Myocarditis presents as heart failure symptoms that develop within days to weeks of an inciting event. It can be preceded by viral prodrome.
- Diagnosis is clinical, and endomyocardial biopsy is indicated in select cases.
- Treatment remains conservative with supportive measures.

CASE 10

Management of Pericardial Effusion Without Cardiac Tamponade

A 43-year-old woman presented to the emergency department with a complaint of worsening shortness of breath for the past 2 days. The patient reported dyspnea on exertion after walking only 2 blocks, when walking upstairs, and sometimes at rest. She complained of chest tightness, which was mainly substernal, 2/10 in intensity, constant, and nonradiating, with no specific aggravating or relieving factors. Additionally, the patient was experiencing orthopnea and paroxysmal nocturnal dyspnea. The patient denied any palpitations, fever, recent travel, sick contacts, or flulike symptoms. Review of systems was otherwise unremarkable. The patient had a past medical history of Hodgkin lymphoma stage IIA treated with chemotherapy 5 years ago and past surgical history of appendectomy. The patient denied the use of tobacco, alcohol, or recreational drugs. No significant family history was reported. She denied taking any medications. On physical examination, vital signs were stable, with blood pressure of 117/70 mm Hg, pulse of 73 bpm, respiratory rate of 17 breaths/min, temperature of 37.1°C (98.8°F), and oxygen saturation of 96% on room air. Physical examination was otherwise unremarkable except for left-sided submandibular lymphadenopathy. Laboratory results showed no acute abnormalities. ECG showed electrical alternans with low-voltage QRS in all limb leads. Chest x-ray showed large mediastinal and hilar lymphadenopathy. Troponin levels were normal. The patient was admitted to the telemetry floor for further monitoring. On the floor, bedside echocardiogram showed moderate pericardial effusion circumferential to the heart with no evidence of hemodynamic compromise or chamber collapse. How would you manage this case?

Case Review

In this case, the patient presented with worsening shortness of breath, chest discomfort, and orthopnea. ECG showed changes of electrical alternans and low-voltage QRS. Chest x-ray showed large mediastinal and hilar lymphadenopathy secondary to Hodgkin lymphoma. In addition, echocardiogram showed moderate pericardial effusion without evidence of tamponade. Based on these data, a diagnosis of pericardial effusion secondary to Hodgkin lymphoma was made, and the cardiology team performed pericardiocentesis to drain the accumulated fluid and sent the fluid for cytology. Cytology was suggestive of malignancy because lymphocytes were predominant. In addition, the surgery team was consulted to create a pericardial window due to the recurrent pericardial effusion.

Case Discussion

Pericardial effusion can develop in patients with acute pericarditis or in association with a variety of systemic diseases. It is characterized by an increased amount of fluid in the pericardial cavity. The most common etiologies of pericardial effusion include malignancy, infection, autoimmune disease, hypothyroidism, and iatrogenic cause (medications, anticoagulation therapy); however, the majority of the cases remain idiopathic. In countries where tuberculosis is endemic, >60% of effusions are caused by tuberculosis.

Clinical Symptoms

Many patients with pericardial effusion are asymptomatic, and the effusion is discovered incidentally with chest radiography or echocardiography. Symptomatic patients present with chest pain, shortness of breath, fatigue, weight loss, and decreased exercise tolerance.

Management

The diagnosis can be suspected from history and findings on ECG and chest imaging. Echocardiogram is required to establish the diagnosis.

   If cancer or bacterial infection is strongly suspected, pericardiocentesis should be considered for diagnostic purposes. In patients with a pericardial effusion of unknown cause and elevated inflammatory markers, empiric treatment of pericarditis may be reasonable. Drainage should be considered if a large idiopathic effusion (>20 mm) is present for >3 months because 1 in 3 patients progress to cardiac tamponade. Treatment is mainly directed toward the etiology of the effusion. Pericardial effusion due to malignancy, tuberculosis, or purulent pericarditis is usually recurrent in nature and requires formation of a pericardial window by surgical or percutaneous balloon dilation. It is a convenient solution to drain fluid in the pleural space where it can be absorbed spontaneously. Use of vasodilators, diuretics, and positive-pressure ventilation should be avoided in order to maintain the preload.

Key Points

- The most common etiologies of pericardial effusion are infection, inflammation, and malignancy.
- Pericardial effusion remains asymptomatic in the majority of the cases.
- Pericardiocentesis is indicated in malignancy, bacterial infection, and large effusions.

7

10 Real Cases on Transient Ischemic Attack and Stroke: Diagnosis, Management, and Follow-Up

Jeirym Miranda • Fareeha S. Alavi • Muhammad Saad

CASE 1

Management of Acute Thrombotic Cerebrovascular Accident Post Recombinant Tissue Plasminogen Activator Therapy

A 59-year-old Hispanic man presented with right upper and lower extremity weakness, associated with facial drop and slurred speech starting 2 hours before the presentation. He denied visual disturbance, headache, chest pain, palpitations, dyspnea, dysphagia, fever, dizziness, loss of consciousness, bowel or urinary incontinence, or trauma. His medical history was significant for uncontrolled type 2 diabetes mellitus, hypertension, hyperlipidemia, and benign prostatic hypertrophy. Social history included cigarette smoking (1 pack per day for 20 years) and alcohol intake of 3 to 4 beers daily. Family history was not significant, and he did not remember his medications. In the emergency department, his vital signs were stable. His physical examination was remarkable for right-sided facial droop, dysarthria, and right-sided hemiplegia. The rest of the examination findings were insignificant. His National Institutes of Health Stroke Scale (NIHSS) score was calculated as 7. Initial CT angiogram of head and neck reported no acute intracranial findings. The neurology team was consulted, and intravenous recombinant tissue plasminogen activator (t-PA) was administered along with high-intensity statin therapy. The patient was admitted to the intensive care unit where his hemodynamics were monitored for 24 hours and later transferred to the telemetry unit. MRI of the head revealed an acute 1.7-cm infarct of the left periventricular white matter and posterior left basal ganglia. How would you manage this case?

Case Review

This case scenario presents a patient with acute ischemic cerebrovascular accident (CVA) requiring intravenous t-PA. Diagnosis was based on clinical neurologic symptoms and an NIHSS score of 7 and was later confirmed by neuroimaging. He had multiple comorbidities, including hypertension, diabetes, dyslipidemia, and smoking history, which put him at a higher risk for developing cardiovascular disease. Because his symptoms started within 4.5 hours of presentation, he was deemed to be a candidate for thrombolytics. The eligibility time line is estimated either by self-report or last witness of baseline status.

Case Discussion

Ischemic strokes are caused by an obstruction of a blood vessel, which irrigates the brain mainly secondary to the development of atherosclerotic changes, leading to cerebral thrombosis and embolism. Diagnosis is made based on presenting symptoms and CT/MRI of the head, and the treatment is focused on cerebral reperfusion based on eligibility criteria and timing of presentation.

Clinical Symptoms

Symptoms include alteration of sensorium, numbness, decreased motor strength, facial drop, dysarthria, ataxia, visual disturbance, dizziness, and headache.

Management

The main goal of thrombotic stroke management is restoration of blood supply to the brain using intravenous thrombolytics. Ensuring a stable airway, breathing, and circulation should be the first step, followed by focused clinical history and neurologic assessment. Intravenous (IV) thrombolytics are indicated within 3 hours of symptom onset with no contraindications. Treatment with t-PA between 3.5 and 4 hours has been used in select group. CT of the head should be performed to exclude hemorrhage, and fingerstick glucose should be checked before administration of t-PA. Although immediate laboratory testing (complete blood count, coagulation panel, cardiac enzymes, and drug toxicology) and ECG can be performed, they should not delay the time to t-PA. Early use of t-PA results in better outcomes and is considered a quality measure in stroke care. The use of stroke scales such as the NIHSS helps to quantify the degree of neurologic deficit and change in clinical status. Blood pressure control with a systolic pressure ≤185 mm Hg and diastolic pressure ≤110 mm Hg should be achieved for at least 24 hours prior to initiating intravenous thrombolytics in those who are eligible. After t-PA use, blood pressure should be maintained at <180/105 mm Hg. All other antithrombotic agents should be kept on hold after 24-hour t-PA until repeat CT of the head rules out intracranial hemorrhage.

Use of t-PA in Stroke

- **Eligibility for t-PA**
  - Age ≥18 years
  - Clinical diagnosis of ischemic stroke causing neurologic deficit
  - Time of symptom onset <4.5 hours
- **Absolute contraindications to t-PA**
  - Intracranial hemorrhage on CT
  - Clinical presentation suggests subarachnoid hemorrhage
  - Neurosurgery, head trauma, or stroke in past 3 months
  - Uncontrolled hypertension (>185 mm Hg systolic or >110 mm Hg diastolic)
  - History of intracranial hemorrhage
  - Known intracranial arteriovenous malformation, neoplasm, or aneurysm

- Active internal bleeding
- Suspected/confirmed endocarditis
- Known bleeding diathesis
- Abnormal blood glucose (<50 mg/dL)
- **Relative contraindications to t-PA**
  - Only minor or rapidly improving stroke symptoms
  - Major surgery or serious nonhead trauma in the previous 14 days
  - History of gastrointestinal or urinary tract hemorrhage within 21 days
  - Seizure at stroke onset
  - Recent arterial puncture at a non-compressible site
  - Recent lumbar puncture
  - Post–myocardial infarction pericarditis
  - Pregnancy
- **Additional warnings to t-PA use >3 hours after stroke**
  - Age >80 years
  - History of prior stroke and diabetes
  - Any active anticoagulant use (even with international normalized ratio <1.7)
  - NIHSS >25
  - CT shows multilobar infarction (hypodensity in greater than one-third of cerebral hemisphere)

Key Points

- Suspect an acute ischemic CVA in a patient with risk factors presenting with neurologic deficit and neuroimaging reporting ischemic changes. Use formal stroke scales such as the NIHSS for clinical and treatment guidance.
- Therapy should include reperfusion therapy in those who are eligible, statins, antiplatelet agents, blood pressure control, and risk factors modification.
- Timing is a determining factor for reperfusion therapy, which is associated with better outcomes, and excluding intracranial hemorrhage must be done prior to any other intervention.

CASE 2

Management of Cardioembolic Stroke

A 69-year-old Hispanic woman was brought to the emergency department for new-onset left-sided facial droop, slurred speech, and left hemiplegia that started 5 hours prior to arrival. She had never experienced these symptoms before. Her medical history included atrial fibrillation, hypertension, hyperlipidemia, and diabetes mellitus. The patient denied any history of smoking, alcohol, or illicit drug use. She mentioned that she does not like to take her medications, which include aspirin, apixaban, lisinopril, and metformin. On presentation, her vital signs were noted to be a blood pressure of 220/113 mm Hg, heart rate of 81 bpm, respiratory rate 16 of breaths/min, and temperature of 98.3°F. On physical examination, she was alert and oriented. Significant neurologic examination included facial asymmetry with nasal fold deviation to the right, dysarthria, and motor strength and sensations severely reduced on the left side and more significantly reduced in the upper extremity. Her National Institutes of Health Stroke Scale (NIHSS) score was calculated as 8. Laboratory data were remarkable for glucose of 315 mg/dL and normal coagulation profile. The initial CT of the head was unremarkable. ECG showed atrial fibrillation with slow ventricular response. She was started on intravenous nicardipine infusion, and rectal aspirin was given. A repeat CT of the head and MRI showed multiple areas of ischemic infarct involving the frontal parietal and occipital areas bilaterally. She was transferred to the telemetry unit. How would you manage this case?

Case Review

This case describes a cardioembolic cause of ischemic stroke. History of atrial fibrillation with nonadherence to anticoagulation is a key here to diagnose the etiology. In addition, the head CT finding of multiple areas of brain involvement bilaterally is another clue toward the diagnosis. In this case, atrial fibrillation is already diagnosed; otherwise, investigation for underlying arrythmia through event monitor should be performed. Echocardiogram should be performed to rule out intracardiac thrombus.

Case Discussion

Embolic stroke is caused by the formation of a thrombus in an artery, vein, heart chamber, or heart valve. It can also be caused by nonthrombotic material such as infected vegetation, valvular calcifications, cardiac tumors (eg, myxoma, papillary fibroelastoma, sarcoma), fibrocartilaginous material, air, or fat. Other emboli can have both thrombotic and non-thrombotic material. Cardioembolic cerebrovascular accidents (CVAs) are associated with a high recurrence rate and poor outcomes compared to other types of CVA.

Clinical Symptoms

Signs and symptoms are similar to those of other types of cerebral vascular disease. However, cardiopulmonary symptoms such as palpitations, chest pain, lightheadedness, and dyspnea may be present.

Management

Management of cardioembolic stroke includes identification of its cause. Arrythmia such as atrial fibrillation is the most commonly associated etiology. Continuous telemetry monitoring using Holter and implantable loop recorder can be performed. Echocardiogram has a pivotal role in recognizing cardiac thrombus and vegetations, with utilization of transesophageal echocardiogram for better assessment of the left atria and ascending aorta. Use of anticoagulation in the setting of atrial fibrillation and intracardiac thrombus has been shown to prevent recurrence. Treatment of the underlying cause should be implemented, along with risk factor control using aspirin, statins, and antihypertensives.

Improvement in stroke recurrence has been observed with use of non–vitamin K antagonist oral anticoagulants in patients with nonvalvular atrial fibrillation. Closure of the left atrial appendage is a nonpharmacologic alternative, especially in patients at higher risk of hemorrhagic stroke, that has shown promising results.

Key Points

- Acute neurologic symptoms with imaging evidence of multiple areas of infarct not limited to a single vessel territory are suspicious for cardioembolic stroke.
- Cardiac arrythmias should be considered in the diagnostic evaluation of ischemic stroke.
- Left ventricular thrombus and valvular vegetations can be identified using echocardiogram.
- Anticoagulation can help prevent recurrent events.

CASE 3

Management of Large-Vessel Stroke

A 52-year-old woman was brought to the hospital by her sister for sudden weakness of her left hand followed by left-sided facial drop and slurring of speech. The symptoms started 6 hours prior to her presentation. She denied fever, trauma, fall, dizziness, and palpitations. Her medical history included hypertension and hyperlipidemia. No relevant family history was found. She admitted use of cocaine 1 week prior and denied alcohol intake or smoking history. On arrival to the emergency department (ED), her vital signs were noted as blood pressure of 126/82 mm Hg, heart rate of 73 bpm, respiratory rate of 16 breaths/min, and temperature of 98.5°F. Physical examination was remarkable for lethargy but ability to follow commands, left nasolabial fold drooping, 1/5 left upper extremity weakness, and 3/5 left lower extremity. The rest of the examination was noncontributory. Stroke code was activated in the ED. National Institutes of Health Stroke Scale (NIHSS) score was 10. Initial CT of the head revealed no evidence of acute intracranial hemorrhage or ischemia. She beyond the window for tissue plasminogen activator because her symptoms started 6 hours prior. Laboratory testing was significant for elevated cardiac enzymes, and drug screen was positive for cocaine and cannabinoids. She was transferred to the telemetry floor. How would you manage this case?

Case Review

This case presents an acute cerebral infarction involving the middle cerebral artery territory. The patient's head MRI showed restricted diffusion with apparent diffusion coefficient (ADC) signal drop-off seen in the right temporoparietal cortex and subcortical white matter consistent with acute middle cerebral artery (MCA) infarction. The patient was beyond the window for thrombolysis and thus was treated with aspirin, high-intensity statin, blood pressure control, and risk factors modification (specifically cocaine cessation) for secondary stroke prevention. Stroke panel consists of head MRI, ultrasound of carotid artery, ECG, echocardiogram, swallow evaluation, and physical therapy.

Case Discussion

The most commonly affected territory in a cerebral infarct is the MCA territory (the parietal lobe, the temporal lobe, and the internal capsule and thalamus), which is related to the area size and its direct flow from the internal carotid artery, leading to the easiest pathway for thromboembolism. MCA infarcts, as opposed to thrombotic infarcts, are generally embolic and typically from the heart or carotid artery. Other risk factors for MCA stroke are similar to those for strokes affecting other locations and include hypertension, hyperlipidemia, diabetes, and cardiac and carotid artery disease.

The development of malignant MCA infarction (extending beyond 50% of the MCA territory) is a life-threatening edema that usually develops 1 to several days after infarction and has a mortality rate of up to 80% in conservatively treated patients.

Clinical Symptoms

Symptoms include contralateral hemiparesis and hemisensory loss, hemianopia, aphasia (expressive [anterior MCA territory infarct], receptive [posterior MCA infarct], or global [extensive infarction]) when affecting the dominant hemisphere, and neglect when the affecting nondominant hemisphere. Early severe neurologic symptoms (hemiparesis, gaze deviation, and higher cortical signs) followed by headache, vomiting, papilledema, and reduced consciousness may predict a malignant course.

Radiologic Findings

CT. CT is useful for predicting the development of malignant brain swelling. The presence of early signs of infarction in a CT implies a worse prognosis.

- Hyperdense MCA sign: Earliest visible sign of MCA infarction seen within 90 minutes after the event; a direct visualization of thromboembolic material within the lumen
- MCA dot sign (Sylvian fissure sign): Represents a thromboembolism within a segmental branch of the MCA located within the Sylvian fissure (M2 segment)
- Insular ribbon sign: Loss of normal gray-white differentiation
- Cortical sulcal effacement
- Obscuration of lentiform nucleus or caudate nucleus: Seen as early as 1 hour after occlusion and visible in 75% of patients at 3 hours
- Large areas of hypodensity (defined as >50% of the MCA territory): Predictive of fatal brain swelling

MRI. MRI demonstrates the typical distribution of affected tissue or occlusion of the vessel, measured by diffusion-weighted imaging or ADC mapping.

Management

Treatment of an MCA infarct is similar to that of infarcts affecting any other territory, with the exception that due to the size of the involved area, which results in space-occupying brain swelling due to vasogenic cerebral edema, patients with malignant MCA stroke are offered decompressive craniectomy as a lifesaving procedure. Osmotic agents (hypertonic saline solutions, mannitol, and glycerol) and steroid therapy are also used to reduce edema and minimize tissue shifts and may be beneficial for bridging to surgical intervention. However, no significant improvement in outcomes has been achieved with these modalities.

Use of stroke scales identifies patients eligible for intravenous thrombolytic or endovascular intervention and those with an elevated risk for complications such as intracerebral hemorrhage. The addition of antithrombotic agents such as aspirin within 48 hours of symptom onset has been shown to reduce complications, disability, and recurrence of stroke. Use of statins in acute stroke management is not supported by evidence.

For patients who are not treated with thrombolytics, blood pressure can be treated in the presence of a systolic or diastolic blood pressure >220 or >120 mm Hg, respectively;

active ischemic coronary disease; aortic dissection; congestive heart failure; hypertensive encephalopathy; or preeclampsia/eclampsia. Fluid management, glucose control, swallowing assessment, physical therapy, and behavioral and lifestyle modifications are important components of stroke care. Management in a stroke unit has been associated with better outcomes.

Key Points

- Large-vessel stroke occurs mainly due to the blockage in carotid vessels with sudden embolization.
- Intravenous thrombolytics should be used if the eligibility criteria are met.
- Risk factor modification, use of antiplatelets, and lipid-lowering therapy should be considered in management.

CASE 4

Management of Transient Ischemic Attack

A 49-year-old woman was brought to the emergency department 45 minutes after she developed slurred speech and numbness and weakness in the right arm that resolved before arriving to the hospital. She denied any headache, blurry vision, palpitations, loss of consciousness, neck pain, or trauma. Her medical history included iron deficiency anemia and hyperlipidemia. Her medications included birth control pills and iron tablets. Family history was not significant for stroke and vascular events. She denied smoking or alcohol or illicit drug use. On arrival, vital signs were noted as blood pressure of 190/100 mm Hg, heart rate of 105 bpm, temperature of 98.8°F, and respiratory rate of 16 breaths/min. Her complete physical examination including neurologic examination was unremarkable. Laboratory testing was significant for moderate microcytic anemia and elevated total cholesterol and low-density lipoprotein levels. Electrolytes, coagulation panel, and drug screen were negative. CT of the head did not show any significant changes. She was transferred to the telemetry floor for further management. How would you manage this case?

Case Review

This case describes a transient ischemic attack (TIA) in a middle-age woman with risk factors including uncontrolled hypertension and hyperlipidemia who presented with neurologic deficits that resolved within 24 hours. The diagnosis of TIA was made after excluding other causes on neuroimaging such as acute cerebrovascular accident, spinal disease, tumors, and multiple sclerosis. The patient was managed conservatively with stroke core measures and risk factor modification.

Case Discussion

TIA is defined as a transient episode of neurologic dysfunction secondary to a focal brain, spinal cord, or retinal ischemia, without acute infarction. Traditionally defined TIA (ie, time based, lasting <24 hours) is associated with a high early risk of recurrent stroke (approximately 4% to 10% in the first 2 days after TIA). The ABCD2 score (Table 7.4.1) was designed to identify patients at high risk of ischemic stroke in this time period, but its predictive performance is not optimal. The diagnosis of TIA (in the absence of tissue infarction) is clinical and based on a determination that the cause of the symptoms is a brain

TABLE 7.4.1 ABCD2 Score	
Age: ≥60 years	1 point
Blood pressure elevation: Systolic ≥140 mm Hg or diastolic ≥90 mm Hg	1 point
Clinical features: Unilateral weakness Isolated speech disturbance	 2 points 1 point
Duration of TIA symptoms: ≥60 minutes 10-59 minutes	 2 points 1 point
Diabetes: Present	1 point

Score interpretation: score of 1 to 3 (low) = 2-day risk of 1.0% and 7-day risk of 1.2%; score of 4 to 5 (moderate) = 2-day risk of 4.1% and 7-day risk of 5.9%; and score of 6 to 7 (high) = 2-day risk of 8.1% and 7-day risk of 11.7%.

ischemia rather than another cause. Diagnosis can be challenging and is usually subjective because the symptoms are transient, often minor, and highly variable.

Clinical Symptoms

The symptoms are similar to those of a stroke, but unlike a stroke, the duration is only a few minutes or hours.

Management

An urgent evaluation is required when TIA is suspected due to the high risk for stroke associated with this entity, which is more closely related to the presence of infarction on diffusion-weighted MRI studies than to the duration of minor neurologic deficit.

According to the American Heart Association and American Stroke Association guidelines, it is reasonable to hospitalize patients with TIA who present within 72 hours of symptom onset and meet any of the following criteria:

- ABCD2 score of ≥3
- ABCD2 score of 0 to 2 and uncertainty that the diagnostic workup can be completed within 2 days as an outpatient
- ABCD2 score of 0 to 2 and other evidence that the event was caused by focal ischemia

The preferred approach to the management of TIA is to determine the etiology and treat accordingly. The initial evaluation includes basic laboratory tests that are suggested by the physical examination and history, neurovascular imaging, and a cardiac evaluation. Laboratory testing is useful in excluding metabolic (hypoglycemia, hyponatremia) and hematologic (thrombocytosis) causes of neurologic symptoms.

Patient should receive immediate stroke prevention with intensive medical therapy that includes antiplatelet or anticoagulant treatment and/or carotid revascularization as appropriate. Those who presents with a potentially disabling persistent neurologic deficit within the appropriate time window after ischemic symptom onset should receive intravenous thrombolysis if not contraindicated despite any degree of improvement. Blood pressure reduction, statin therapy, and lifestyle modification including smoking cessation are the mainstay for secondary stroke prevention.

Key Points

- TIA is defined as an acute neurologic deficit that resolves within 24 hours.
- The ABCD2 score can be used to identify patients at high risk for recurrent events.
- Management includes aggressive risk factor control and stroke care.

CASE 5

Management of Feeding Issues After Stroke

A 73-year-old man was brought to the hospital by his daughter for inability to eat since he had a stroke diagnosed 1 month earlier. At the time of his hospital discharge, he was able to eat chopped food but had subsequently been unable to do it for 2 weeks. At presentation, he did not have any fever, urinary symptoms, cough, blurry vision, or respiratory symptoms. His medical history included hypertension, diabetes mellitus, hyperlipidemia, dementia, and recent middle cerebral artery (MCA) territory cerebrovascular accident (CVA) with right-sided residual weakness and facial asymmetry. He lived with his daughter who indicated the patient had poor oral intake causing significant weight loss and difficulty taking medications. No significant family history or social history was noted. In the emergency department, the patient's vital signs were stable, and he was alert and oriented to time, place, and person. Physical examination was significant for right-sided weakness greater in the arm than leg and difficulty in speaking sentences. CT of the head showed left frontal area ischemic stroke with stable changes. The patient was transferred to the telemetry floor for further management. What kind of care will you provide to this patient?

Case Review

The case describes an elderly male patient diagnosed with acute MCA territory stroke with residual neurologic dysfunction that has severely affected his ability to function independently. Stroke has been associated with several complications, among which feeding is a main issue. Poor nutrition puts stroke patient at risk of aspiration pneumonia, malnourishment, and other opportunistic infections, resulting in higher morbidity and mortality. Goals of care should be identified in collaboration with the patient and healthcare proxy. There are various options that should be discussed with patient and family that can serve as a temporary or long-term feeding support.

Case Discussion

On initial presentation of a stroke patient, independent predictors of dysphagia include disabling stroke, male sex, age >70 years, impaired pharyngeal response, incomplete oral clearance, and palatal weakness or asymmetry.

In stroke care, it is essential for appropriately trained staff to screen and assess for swallowing problems in all patients after an acute stroke before they are given any oral food, fluid, or medication. It is also recommended that if there is any evidence of swallowing difficulty, then the swallow assessment should take place within 24 hours after admission. This has been shown to be was associated with a significantly decreased risk of aspiration pneumonia.

Prevention of aspiration includes initial nil per os (NPO) status for those who failed the swallow test and are unable to safely tolerate oral fluids or food. Nasogastric tube (NGT) should be placed for temporary provision of nutrition and hydration within 24 hours. If patient is unable to tolerate an NGT, then a nasal bridle or a gastrostomy tube should be considered, while efforts are made to restore swallowing.

The prevalence of malnutrition after an acute CVA ranges from 8% to 34%, and most patients with dysphagia recover within the first 4 weeks; however, 15% of patients develop long-term swallowing dysfunction. Although 20% of patients may require enteral tube feeding during the acute phase after a stroke, 8% will require long-term enteral tube feeding for >6 months.

There are variety of enteral feeding tubes. Short-term interventions include insertion of an NGT, whereas long-term nutritional support involves insertion of a percutaneous endoscopic gastrostomy (PEG) tube.

Important considerations concerning enteral and parenteral feeding include the following:

- Begin early enteral feeding (ie, within 48 hours) in patients without contraindications to enteral nutrition. During the first 5 to 7 days of critical illness, do not exceed 20% to 30% of the feeding goal, unless the patient is quite stable.
- Do not initiate early parenteral nutrition, and typically do not start feeding parenterally before 1 to 2 weeks have elapsed in adequately nourished patients who have contraindications or intolerance to enteral nutrition. This reflects the evidence that early parenteral nutrition may increase the risk of infection and prolong mechanical ventilation, intensive care unit stay, and hospital stay.
- Parenteral nutrition can be initiated before 1 to 2 weeks have elapsed in patients with antecedent starvation and/or wasting who have contraindications to enteral nutrition that are expected to persist for a week or more. Supplemental parenteral nutrition may be administered to patients receiving enteral nutrition but who are chronically unable to meet their needs by a significant margin.
- For obese patients (body mass index ≥30 kg/m^2), it is recommended to use the same indications for enteral and parenteral nutrition as for the adequately nourished critically ill patient. The chronically starved and/or wasted but still obese patient is likely to be more ill and at higher risk for complications related to undernourishment.

Complications of enteral and parenteral nutrition include the following:

- Enteral nutrition: The most common complications are aspiration, diarrhea, metabolic abnormalities, and mechanical complications.
- Parenteral nutrition: The most common complications are bloodstream infection, metabolic abnormalities, and problems related to venous access.

Key Points
- Feeding issues are a major complication of large-vessel stroke and are associated with higher morbidity and mortality.
- Evaluation for swallowing should be initiated within 24 hours.
- Short-term and long-term feeding methods should be used while natural recovery occurs.

CASE 6

Management of Intracerebral Hemorrhage

A 55-year-old man was brought to the emergency department (ED) with complaints of headache and blurry vision for 12 hours that started suddenly and were not relieved by acetaminophen. The symptoms were associated with nausea and 1 episode of nonbloody vomiting. He was in his usual state of health 1 day prior with full activity. He denied any trauma, history of headache in the past, runny nose, jaw claudication, dizziness, fever, or loss of consciousness. His medical history included hypertension, severe mitral valve regurgitation, and recent right popliteal deep vein thrombosis (DVT). He denied any toxic habits and any significant family history. Medications included warfarin, lisinopril, and furosemide. In the ED, his vital signs were stable and fingerstick glucose was normal. Urgent CT of the head was done, which showed a small intraparenchymal bleed. Laboratory tests were significant for an international normalized ratio of 5; cell count and electrolytes were normal. Neurology, neurosurgery, and hematology teams were consulted. No acute neurosurgical intervention was recommended. The intensive care unit staff evaluated the patient and decided to admit him on the telemetry floor based on stable hemodynamics. Anticoagulation and antiplatelet therapy were placed on hold. Vitamin K and fresh frozen plasma were administered. How would you manage this case?

Case Review

This patient was diagnosed with acute intracerebral hemorrhage (ICH) in the setting of use of anticoagulation for acute DVT. This case describes a common but catastrophic complication of the use of anticoagulation in patient with thromboembolic disease. Reversal of anticoagulation should be performed with frequent monitoring of neurologic assessment and blood pressure control. Repeat imaging should be performed if symptoms deteriorate to assess for cerebral edema and midline shift, which is a sign of a neurosurgical emergency. A small stable bleed can be managed conservatively. Seizure prophylaxis can be initiated with a large bleed, guided by expert opinion.

Case Discussion

ICH is the second most frequent cause of cerebrovascular accident (9% to 27% of all strokes globally) after ischemic stroke. ICH affects 12 to 31 per 100,000 people, with a higher incidence in Asians, intermediate incidence in blacks, and the lowest incidence in whites. There are many underlying pathologic conditions associated with ICH, and the majority of cases include hypertensive vasculopathy (most common), ruptured saccular aneurysm, amyloid angiopathy (the most common cause of nontraumatic lobar ICH in older adults), and vascular malformation (in children). Other causes include hemorrhagic infarction, septic embolism, mycotic aneurysm, brain tumor, bleeding disorders, liver disease, thrombolytic therapy, and drugs (eg, cocaine, amphetamines).

Clinical Symptoms

The signs and symptoms of ICH will vary according to the size and location of hemorrhage. The presenting neurologic deficit is acute in onset and usually increases gradually over minutes or a few hours. Headache, vomiting, and a decreased level of consciousness are the presenting symptoms. If intraventricular hemorrhage develops, neck stiffness and meningismus can be found on physical examination. Seizures occur in 15% of cases, especially if the hemorrhage is located superficially.

Management

ICH is a medical emergency due to the high risk of ongoing bleeding, progressive neurologic deterioration, permanent disability, and death. Management should be provided in an intensive care unit or dedicated stroke unit with expertise in neurology, neurosurgery, neuroradiology, and critical care. To confirm the diagnosis of ICH and to exclude ischemic stroke and other causes, it is essential to perform neuroimaging with CT/MRI of the head.

Acute interventions include airway protection with intubation and mechanical ventilation, discontinuation of all anticoagulant and antiplatelet medication, anticoagulation reversal with appropriate agents, blood pressure control, intracranial pressure (ICP) monitoring, aspiration precautions with repeated swallow evaluation, seizure prophylaxis, and glycemic control. Surgical options include ventriculostomy and hematoma evacuation. The most important step to prevent hematoma-associated neurologic complications is to control blood pressure. Other risk factor modifications including cessation of smoking, heavy alcohol use, and illicit drug use.

- Blood pressure management: Target blood pressure range is a systolic blood pressure of 140 to 160 mm Hg. Aggressive reduction can be done using a continuous intravenous infusion of antihypertensive medication such as labetalol.
- Elevated ICP management: Elevate the head of the bed to 30 degrees, provide mild sedation, and use normal saline for maintenance and replacement fluids. Other aggressive measures to decrease ICP include osmotic diuretics (mannitol or hypertonic saline), neuromuscular blockade, pharmacologic coma, hyperventilation, and ventricular drainage of cerebrospinal fluid.
- Surgical removal of hemorrhage: This is recommended for patients with cerebellar hemorrhages >3 cm in diameter or for cerebellar hemorrhage patients with deteriorating neurologic status or who have brainstem compression and/or hydrocephalus due to ventricular obstruction. It is also reserved for patients with life-threatening mass effect from supratentorial ICH, based on individual assessment of prognosis.

Key Points

- ICH can be associated with hypertensive vasculopathy, amyloid angiopathy, subarachnoid hemorrhage, and arteriovenous malformation.
- Presenting symptoms include headache, vomiting, and signs of meningismus.
- Urgent CT of the head should be performed for diagnosis.
- Management includes blood pressure control and monitoring of ICP with timely surgical intervention, if needed.

CASE 7

Management of Migraine With Brainstem Aura

A 29-year-old woman was brought to the emergency department (ED) reporting confusion and occipital headache for the past 2 hours that were associated with nausea, dizziness, blurry vision, and perioral tingling. She had 2 similar episodes in the past, which she noticed were associated with emotional stress. She denied gait instability, loss of consciousness, ear discharge, fever, weakness, and numbness. There was no significant medical history or family history. She denied taking any medications or using alcohol, tobacco, or illicit drugs. On arrival to ED, vitals were stable. Physical examination, including neurologic examination, was noncontributory. Routine laboratory tests were within normal limits. CT of the head did not show any acute findings. She was given ketorolac injection and transferred to the telemetry floor. How would you manage this case?

Case Review

This young woman with no risk factors for transient ischemic attack (TIA)/stroke should be evaluated for basilar migraine. Usually detailed clinical history can exclude many differential diagnoses. The basic workup includes head CT, ECG, and electrolyte panel. MRI of the head can show nonspecific changes. Because of the of lack of significant risk factors and normal laboratory testing and neuroimaging in this patient, other causes of her symptoms are less likely. Analgesics such as nonsteroidal anti-inflammatory drugs can provide complete symptom relief. Differential diagnosis includes TIA, psychogenic attacks or behavioral spells, Ménière disease, brain tumor, Chiari malformation, familial or sporadic hemiplegic migraine, temporal lobe epilepsy/complex partial seizures, basilar aneurysm, subarachnoid hemorrhage, benign paroxysmal positional vertigo, acute labyrinthitis, and tumors of the posterior fossa.

Case Discussion

Migraine with brainstem aura (MBA), previously called basilar-type migraine, is a rare form of migraine with aura where the primary signs and symptoms seem to originate from the brainstem, without evidence of weakness. There is no evidence that the basilar artery is involved, because some of the symptoms may localize outside the territory of the basilar artery. MBA has no predilection for any age or sex, with a female-to-male ratio ranging from 1.3:1 to 3.8:1. The difference between MBA and migraine with typical aura is that the location of the aura symptoms in MBA primarily involves the brainstem or the bilateral occipital hemispheres, whereas in typical migraine, the aura symptoms are mainly restricted to a unilateral hemisphere. Migraine can be triggered by emotional stress, menstruation, head trauma, food, contraceptive drugs, smoking, exertion, and pressure changes.

Clinical Symptoms

Symptoms include unilateral or bilateral hemianopia, ataxia, vertigo, dysarthria, bilateral tingling, or numbness. The aura is usually followed by a throbbing occipital headache and nausea. Loss of consciousness lasting 2 to 30 minutes can occur in 25% of patients. The paroxysmal nature of the symptoms and their complete resolution and strong family and personal history of migraine are characteristic of MBA.

The diagnostic criteria for MBA are as follows:

A) At least 2 attacks fulfilling criteria B through D	**B)** Aura consisting of visual, sensory, and/or speech/language symptoms, each fully reversible, but no motor or retinal symptoms
C) At least 2 of the following brainstem symptoms: • Dysarthria • Vertigo • Tinnitus • Hyperacusis • Diplopia • Ataxia • Decreased level of consciousness	**D)** At least 2 of the following 4 characteristics: • At least 1 aura symptom spreads gradually over ≥5 minutes, and/or 2 or more symptoms occur in succession. • Each individual aura symptom lasts 5–60 minutes. • At least 1 aura symptom is unilateral. • The aura is accompanied, or followed within 60 minutes, by headache.
E) Transient ischemic attack has been excluded	

Data from the International Classification of Headache Disorders, Third Edition (ICHD-3).

Management

MBA is diagnosed by focused history and physical examination with no specific diagnostic test. Treatment of MBA is similar to that for migraine with typical aura and common migraine, except agents that may theoretically cause or exacerbate ischemia (β-blockers, triptans, or ergotamine derivatives) should be avoided.

- Acute therapy: Antiemetics such as phenothiazine and other nonvasoconstricting abortive agents such as nonsteroidal anti-inflammatory drugs.
- Preventive therapy: Initial treatment with either sustained-release verapamil or topiramate for patients with frequent, prolonged, or debilitating attacks. Treatment with lamotrigine is suggested for those who fail to benefit from verapamil or topiramate and for those with persistent aura symptoms that predominate over headache.

Key Points

- Basilar migraine or MBA should be considered in evaluation of TIA and cerebellar stroke when conventional risk factors for these events are not present.
- Workup includes exclusion of organic causes.
- Treatment strategy includes abortive and preventive therapy.

CASE 8

Management of Vertebral Artery Dissection

A 54-year-old man presented to the hospital after a 5-hour history of gradual left-sided arm and facial weakness followed by sudden onset of severe neck pain and occipital headache. He denied fever, blurry vision, gait problems, urinary or bowel issues, and tingling or numbness. Medical history was significant for hypertension. He denied any toxic habits or significant family history. He reported having a motor vehicle accident 2 weeks ago with minor abrasions on his chest and back for which he went to a local emergency department

(ED) and received treatment. Because his pain was not getting better, he received chiropractic treatment, which did not help. On arrival to the ED, he was alert and oriented and hemodynamically stable, with a blood pressure of 156/78 mm Hg, heart rate of 80 bpm, and respiratory rate of 18 breaths/min. Physical examination was significant for decreased motor strength on the right upper extremity and scalp tenderness. Funduscopic examination was unremarkable. CT of the head did not show any significant findings. A basic laboratory panel was normal. Because he was beyond the time window for tissue plasminogen activator (t-PA), he received aspirin and a statin and was sent to the telemetry floor for stroke workup. On the telemetry floor, he developed worsening of weakness on the right side, along with vertigo, nausea, and vomiting. An emergent CT angiogram of the head and neck was done that showed a right occipital area infarct with reduced flow in the right vertebral artery with a dissection flap, consistent with right vertebral artery dissection. How would you manage this case?

Case Review

This patient was diagnosed with acute ischemic cerebrovascular accident (CVA) secondary to right vertebral artery dissection likely following minor traumatic injury due to the motor vehicle accident and chiropractic manipulation. His presenting symptoms are typical of those seen in this disease, and treatment with an intravenous thrombolytic or anticoagulation and antiplatelet therapy should be initiated. Vascular surgery or interventional radiology should also be consulted for endovascular repair. Frequent neurologic assessment can be performed in a monitored setting. Avoidance of sudden or excessive neck manipulation or sports involving neck motion is recommended.

Case Discussion

Spontaneous dissection is a common cause of stroke, accounting for approximately 20% of ischemic CVAs. It commonly affects young adults but may occur at any age, with the mean age between 44 and 46 years.

Major head and neck trauma is associated with vertebral artery dissection, but most dissections occur spontaneously after trivial or nonserious injury (vigorous exercise; physical activities such as skating, tennis, basketball, volleyball, swimming, scuba diving, or dancing; or roller coaster or amusement park rides). Other reported precipitating activities include childbirth, sexual intercourse, coughing or sneezing, and chiropractic neck manipulation.

Various connective tissue and vascular disorders are associated with vertebral artery dissection, including fibromuscular dysplasia, Ehlers-Danlos syndrome type IV, Marfan syndrome, osteogenesis imperfects, homocystinuria, autosomal dominant polycystic kidney disease, α_1-antitrypsin deficiency, reticular fiber deficiency, segmental mediolytic arteriopathy, cystic medial necrosis, reversible cerebral vasoconstriction syndromes, and cervical artery tortuosity.

Vertebral artery dissection most commonly affects the V3 segment at the C1 to C2 level.

Clinical Symptoms

Neurologic complications may result from ischemic stroke or transient ischemic attack due to thromboembolism (major cause), hypoperfusion, or a combination of both. In addition, dissection and aneurysmal dilatation can cause local symptoms from compression of adjacent nerves and their feeding vessels, producing neck or head pain (first initial symptoms) or thunderclap headache and partial oculosympathetic paresis (Horner syndrome involving ptosis and miosis but not anhidrosis; seen in 25% of cases with internal carotid artery dissection). Other manifestations include tinnitus, an audible bruit, lower cranial neuropathies, scalp tenderness, cervical nerve root involvement (a rare complication of vertebral artery dissection), and isolated orbital or monocular pain (rare presentation of carotid artery dissection).

Management

Although clinical features may raise suspicion for dissection, the diagnosis is confirmed with MRI and magnetic resonance angiography of the brain and neck or cranial CT with CT angiogram. The characteristic imaging findings are string sign, intimal flap, long tapered stenosis or occlusion or flame-shaped occlusion, distal pouch, a double lumen, and a dissecting aneurysm (pseudoaneurysm). A pathognomonic crescent sign, formed by an eccentric rim of hyperintensity surrounding a hypointense arterial lumen, on MRI signifies underlying arteriopathy and intramural hematoma.

Treatment with thrombolytic therapy in very early acute ischemic stroke should not be delayed for eligible patients. After the hyperacute period, either anticoagulation or antiplatelet medications can be used to treat ischemic stroke and transient ischemic attack caused by extracranial vertebral artery dissection. The use of thrombolytics and antithrombotic agents in patients with intracranial dissection alone or intracranial extension of extracranial dissection is controversial because of the presumed increased risk of subarachnoid hemorrhage.

Antithrombotic treatment must be held until 24 hours after thrombolytic administration. Anticoagulants can be initiated in patients who are not treated with intravenous thrombolytic therapy. Treatment with antiplatelet therapy is suggested for primary prevention of ischemic stroke in patients with nonischemic symptoms caused by extracranial vertebral artery dissection, and headache and neck pain can be managed with simple analgesia.

Endovascular methods and mechanical surgical repair have been used to treat dissection with recurrent ischemia despite antithrombotic therapy and to treat intracranial dissection with subarachnoid hemorrhage.

The prognosis is related to the severity of ischemic stroke or subarachnoid hemorrhage. In patients with extracranial dissection, recovery occurs in 70% to 85%, disabling deficits occur in 10% to 25%, and death occurs in 5% to 10%. However, in patients with intracranial dissection, morbidity and mortality rates are higher.

Key Points

- Vertebral artery dissection can be spontaneous or secondary to trauma.
- Symptoms include headache, focal deficit, nausea, vomiting, vertigo, diplopia, and cerebellar symptoms.
- Antiplatelet agents or anticoagulants should be used for treatment.

CASE 9

Management of Cerebellar Stroke

A 68-year-old man was brought to the emergency department (ED) by his daughter with a complaint of intermittent episodes of dizziness for 2 days. The dizziness was described as a room spinning sensation associated with nausea and 1 episode of vomiting. He reported unsteady gait with the tendency to fall toward the right side. The symptoms had been gradually becoming more frequent since the day before presentation without any specific aggravating or alleviating factors. He denied fever, neck pain, headache, palpitations, weakness, or numbness. His medical history included hypertension, type 2 diabetes mellitus, hyperlipidemia, and gastroesophageal reflux disease. The patient was a smoker who smoked 1 pack of cigarettes daily for the past 30 years. He denied any alcohol or illicit drug use. There was no significant family history. His medications included metformin, omeprazole, simvastatin, and lisinopril. On arrival to the ED, he was alert and oriented to person, time, and space; his vital signs were stable; and he had negative orthostatic vitals. Physical examination was remarkable for horizontal nystagmus in the right eye and truncal ataxia. Gait could not be assessed due to persistent dizziness. Dysdiadochokinesia was also noted. Laboratory testing was significant for elevated low-density lipoprotein and hemoglobin A1c of 9%. CT of the head did not show any acute changes. He was given aspirin and a statin and transferred to the telemetry floor for further stroke workup. How would you manage this case?

Case Review

This patient has risk factors for cerebrovascular stroke. Dizziness with nystagmus and gait instability should be evaluated for cerebellar stroke. Because the pretest probability for cerebrovascular accident (CVA) is high, negative CT of the head does not exclude the diagnosis. The patient should get an MRI of the head for detailed evaluation of posterior fossa structures. Cerebellar strokes can be associated with herniation; therefore, frequent neurologic checks should be performed. Blood pressure control and antiplatelet medications should be initiated.

When evaluating a patient with similar complaints, the differential diagnosis can also include vestibular neuronitis, migraine, hypertensive emergency, benign paroxysmal positional vertigo, syncope (vasovagal, orthostatic, or arrhythmic), hypoglycemia, and ethanol or drug intoxication.

Case Discussion

Cerebellar infarction is a relatively rare subtype of ischemic stroke, accounting for approximately 2% of all cerebral infarcts. It occurs in patients with risk factors such as hypertension, diabetes, and old age (>60 years). The most common causes are atherosclerosis, embolism, and dissection involving any of the 3 arteries supplying the cerebellum (superior cerebellar artery [SCA], anterior inferior cerebellar artery [AICA], and posterior inferior cerebellar artery [PICA; most frequent location]). Although cerebellar stroke composes a small fraction of strokes, its morbidity and mortality are higher than other types of stroke. This is generally due to concomitant brainstem infarction, reactive edema leading to upward transtentorial herniation of the cerebellar vermis, or obstruction of the fourth ventricle and aqueducts anteriorly, causing direct brainstem compression with herniation of the cerebellar tonsils into the foramen magnum.

Clinical Symptoms

In contrast to cerebral strokes, neurologic findings in cerebellar stroke are usually ipsilesional. Symptoms are usually more severe than examination findings and are governed by the involved vascular territories. Dizziness with a sensation of vertigo or of falling toward one side is reported in 75% of cases, and nausea or vomiting is reported in >50% of cases. From rostral to caudal, symptoms of cerebellar strokes include the following:

- SCA infarct: Can cause more ataxia, dysarthria, and nystagmus, with less vertigo, headache, and vomiting.
- AICA infarct: Dysmetria, Horner syndrome, unilateral hearing loss, and ipsilateral facial paralysis or anesthesia with contralateral hemibody sensory loss of pain and temperature.
- PICA infarct: Headache and less commonly vomiting, vertigo, horizontal ipsilateral nystagmus, and truncal ataxia. Full PICA territory infarcts are often accompanied by edema formation and mass effect (called pseudotumoral cerebellar infarction). Bilateral Babinski signs are an early sign of cerebellar mass effect.
- Lethargy, frank coma, or cardiovascular collapse is seen in patients with larger strokes or with advanced features of elevated intracranial pressure or brainstem compression, which portend a poor outcome.

Management

Cerebellar infarcts are treated similar to ischemic CVA, with risk stratification and treatment planning determined by clinical findings. Besides focused history and physical examination, supportive testing includes neuroimaging such as MRI of the brain. Furthermore, ECG, echocardiographic, and electroencephalographic evaluation for other systemic conditions should be obtained to assist with concurrent medical or surgical management.

MRI with diffusion-weighted imaging (DWI) of the brain is the gold standard test for cerebellar infarction. A CT scan can exclude cerebellar hemorrhage and should be done urgently if MRI is not immediately available.

Thrombolysis with recombinant tissue plasminogen activator (rt-PA) may be given when there is a clear time of onset within 4.5 hours and if there are no contraindication. However, this is often not possible given the difficulty of diagnosing posterior infarcts. In the presence of a large difference or "mismatch" between the volume of brain infarcted and the area of decreased perfusion or a high degree of collateral circulation seen on neuroimaging, thrombectomy can be an option. Treatment with aspirin and possibly another antiplatelet agent such as clopidogrel is indicated when reperfusion is not an option. The addition of anticoagulation therapy should be considered in patients with embolic events.

Reactive cerebral edema usually worsens 3 to 4 days after the initial infarct, causing worsening neurologic symptoms, especially if intracranial pressure is elevated, and often requires extraventricular drains, ventriculostomy, or decompressive suboccipital craniotomy. In the acute setting, mannitol, hypertonic saline, or hyperventilation can also be helpful to temporarily reduce intracranial pressure. Physical therapy has a key role in gait training and rehabilitation.

Key Points

- Cerebellar stroke presents with dizziness, nausea, vomiting, and gait instability.
- Thorough clinical examination with assessment of cerebellar signs should be performed, followed by imaging such as MRI of the brain.
- Treatment includes routine stroke care along with frequent neurologic assessments for worsening signs of herniation.

CASE 10

Management of Lacunar Stroke

A 71-year-old woman presented to the emergency department (ED) accompanied by her husband with complaints of left-sided numbness of the face and left arm. Symptoms started 8 hours prior and remained persistent. She denied weakness, fever, neck pain, vision problem, headache, nausea, vomiting, and urinary and bowel issues. Her medical history included uncontrolled hypertension, hyperlipidemia, and transient ischemic attack (TIA). She was a former smoker and quit 20 years ago. She denied any alcohol or illicit drug use. No significant family history was noted. She had been able to perform her activities of daily living. On arrival to the ED, vital signs were noted as blood pressure of 170/93 mm Hg, heart rate of 69 bpm, and respiratory rate of 18 breaths/min. On physical examination, she was alert and oriented, with no significant neurologic deficit except decreased sensation to touch and pain on the left side of her face and arm. Laboratory tests, including cell counts, electrolytes, cholesterol, low-density lipoprotein, and thyroid panel, were within normal limits. Drug screening test was also negative. CT of the head showed no acute findings. She was treated with aspirin and a statin and transferred to the telemetry floor for further stroke workup. How would you manage this case?

Case Review

Sensory symptoms in a patient with conventional risk factors for stroke should be considered with caution. Although head CT can be negative, the diagnosis should be confirmed with MRI brain. Aggressive control of risk factors and physical therapy are key in management. Cardioembolic causes should be evaluated by ECG and echocardiographic testing. This patient had a brain MRI that showed a right thalamic lacunar infarct.

Case Discussion

Lacunar infarcts are small noncortical infarct (0.2 to 15 mm in diameter) that are caused by the obstruction of a single penetrating branch of a large cerebral artery and account for 15% to 26% of all ischemic strokes. These branches originate at acute angles from the large arteries of the circle of Willis, the stem of the middle cerebral artery, and the basilar artery. The most common locations affected by lacunar infarct are the basal ganglia (putamen, globus pallidus, thalamus, and caudate), subcortical white matter (internal capsule and corona radiata), and pons.

The mechanism of lacunar infarct is related to a chronic vasculopathy associated with systemic hypertension. Other risk factors include diabetes mellitus, elevated low-density lipoprotein cholesterol, and smoking.

Clinical Symptoms

Penetrating artery occlusion typically causes symptoms that develop over a short period of time, usually minutes to hours. However, it can evolve over several days, similar to large artery thrombosis. In general, lacunar syndromes are characterized by the absence of "cortical" signs, such as neglect, apraxia, aphasia, agnosia, or hemianopsia. Monoplegia, stupor, coma, loss of consciousness, and seizures are also absent.

Classic lacunar syndromes include the following:

- Pure motor hemiparesis: Most frequent, affecting 45% to 57%. Described as unilateral paralysis of face, arm, and leg in the absence of sensory or cortical deficits. Location is usually at the internal capsule, corona radiata, basal pons, or medial medulla.
- Pure sensory stroke: Seen in 7% to 18% of lacunar syndromes. Defined as numbness of the face, arm, and leg on one side of the body without motor deficits. Thalamus, pontine tegmentum, and corona radiate are the affected locations.
- Ataxic hemiparesis: Consistent with unilateral weakness and limb ataxia and seen in 3% to 18% of lacunar syndromes. Dysarthria, nystagmus, and gait deviation toward the affected side may be present in some patients. Infarction is typically located on the internal capsule–corona radiata, basal pons, or thalamus.
- Sensorimotor stroke: Hemiparesis or hemiplegia of face, arm, and leg with ipsilateral sensory impairment. Responsible for 15% to 20% of lacunar syndromes. Affects the thalamocapsular area, basal pons, or lateral medulla.
- Dysarthria–clumsy hand syndrome: This is the least common type and accounts for 2% to 6% of lacunar syndromes. It is defined by unilateral facial weakness, dysarthria, and dysphagia, with mild hand weakness and clumsiness. The basal pons, internal capsule, and corona radiate are commonly affected areas.

Management

The diagnosis of lacunar infarct is based on the presence of a clinical syndrome that is consistent with the location of a small noncortical infarct seen on CT or MRI. Brain imaging with CT or MRI is also helpful to exclude other potentially life-threatening diagnoses such as intracerebral hemorrhage or subdural hematoma.

As opposed to ischemic stroke in general, no proven treatment has shown benefit specifically for lacunar infarction. The main goal in the acute management is to ensure medical stability, to evaluate the pathophysiologic basis of the neurologic symptoms, and to determine the eligibility for thrombolysis, which showed better outcomes in lacunar stroke.

Treatment with aspirin should be initiated in patients who are not eligible for thrombolytic therapy. The major focus of treatment should be on secondary prevention with intensive medical treatment and risk factor modification, including antihypertensive, antiplatelet, and statin therapy. Smoking cessation counseling and physical therapy should be part of the management protocol.

Key Points

- Lacunar stroke is a type of ischemic stroke caused by occlusion of small penetrating branches of large arteries of the brain.
- It is common in patient with uncontrolled hypertension, patients with hyperlipidemia, smokers, and diabetics.
- Common locations of the brain involved are the basal ganglia and subcortical white matter structures.
- Aggressive control of risk factors is the key in management.

8

10 Real Cases on Peripheral Artery Disease and Carotid Artery Disease: Diagnosis, Management, and Follow-Up

Niel Shah • Muhammad Ameen • Muhammad Saad

CASE 1

Management of Progressive Peripheral Arterial Disease Despite Initial Medical Management

A 65-year-old man was sent from the clinic for worsening of left calf severe pain and decrease in exercise tolerance due to left calf pain. The patient had a 3-month history of intermittent left calf pain and denied trauma, back pain, fever, and leg weakness. Otherwise, the medical history was significant for hyperlipidemia. He was a former smoker and stopped smoking 6 months ago; however, he smoked 1 pack of cigarettes per day for the past 40 years before quitting. The patient denied use of alcohol or recreational drugs. His medications were low-dose aspirin and high-intensity atorvastatin. On physical examination, vital signs were normal. Body mass index was 28 kg/m². Femoral pulses were diminished bilaterally. Popliteal, right dorsalis pedis, and right posterior tibialis pulses were faint. The left dorsalis pedis and posterior tibialis pulses were not palpable. Cardiac examination was normal. Otherwise, the physical examination was unremarkable. The ankle-brachial index was 0.67 on the left and 0.91 on the right. He was enrolled in a supervised exercise program 3 months ago, but the patient reported no improvement despite adherence to the exercise program, and his symptoms progressed. How would you manage this case?

Case Review

This scenario represents a patient with progressive peripheral arterial disease (PAD) despite being on initial medical management. The signs of progressive PAD include progressive decrease in exercise tolerance due to worsening left leg pain and physical examination findings of nonpalpable dorsalis pedis and posterior tibialis pulse on the left side. The patient

129

is already on initial medical management of PAD, including smoking cessation, aspirin, high-intensity statins, and a supervised exercise program.

Case Discussion

PAD is most commonly characterized by narrowing of the aortic bifurcation and arteries of the lower extremities, including the iliac, femoral, popliteal, and tibial arteries. Atherosclerosis is the most common cause. Risk factors for PAD include smoking (current or past), diabetes mellitus, and increasing age. Patients with PAD are at increased risk for ischemic events, including myocardial infarction, stroke, and cardiovascular death. Patients with atherosclerotic risk factors (smoking, diabetes, hypertension, dyslipidemia, and advanced age) who have atypical limb symptoms (eg, leg weakness, paresthesia), exertional leg discomfort, and/or nonhealing ulcers should undergo initial testing with ankle-brachial index (ABI) measurement.

Clinical Symptoms

There is a wide spectrum of clinical manifestations because lower extremity PAD is defined by an abnormal ABI value rather than by symptoms. Patients may present with exertional leg pain relieved by rest (intermittent claudication), atypical exertional leg pain, rest pain, nonhealing wounds, ischemic ulcers, or gangrene.

ABI interpretation is as follows:

- ABI 0.00 to 0.40: Severe PAD
- ABI 0.41 to 0.90: Mild to moderate PAD
- ABI 0.91 to 0.99: Borderline PAD
- ABI 1.00 to 1.40: Normal
- ABI >1.40: Noncompressible (calcified) vessel (uninterpretable result)

Management

Initial medical management of PAD includes risk factor modifications, such as smoking cessation, high-intensity statins, diabetes control, and blood pressure control. In addition, patients should be started on antiplatelet therapy, such as aspirin, to decrease the risk of myocardial infarctions, stroke, and peripheral arterial events. Furthermore, patients should be encouraged to enroll in the supervised exercise program, which can improve symptoms. This patient is already on the initial medical management of PAD; thus, the most appropriate next step in management is to initiate cilostazol (a phosphodiesterase inhibitor with antiplatelet and vasodilator activity). The US Food and Drug Administration has placed a black box warning on the use of cilostazol in patients with heart failure. In patients with intermittent claudication and confirmed lower extremity PAD with an abnormal ABI (≤0.9), exercise training and medical therapy (cilostazol) have been shown to improve limb symptoms. If this patient does not have improvement in his symptoms with cilostazol or cannot tolerate cilostazol therapy, he should be referred for invasive management (endovascular or surgical revascularization).

Key Points

- Patients with symptomatic PAD may present with exertional leg pain relieved by rest (intermittent claudication), atypical exertional leg pain, rest pain, nonhealing wounds, ischemic ulcers, or gangrene.

- Medical management, such as risk modification, antithrombotics, exercise training, and pharmacologic therapy (cilostazol), is recommended to improve limb symptoms in patients with PAD and intermittent claudication.

CASE 2

Management of Pseudoclaudication

A 70-year-old woman presented to the emergency department with cramping pain in the buttocks and thighs with standing and walking. Symptoms were exacerbated after standing at work for several hours and were relieved by sitting. The patient reported she had been having these symptoms for the past 6 to 8 months and they were stable. However, recently she started noticing worsening of the symptoms. She denied trauma, focal deficit, and loss of sphincteric control. Her past medical history was significant for hypertension. She did not report a history of any major surgery. She smoked cigarettes for many years but stopped smoking 12 years ago. She denied alcohol use or intravenous or recreational drug use. Her home medications were amlodipine and lisinopril. On physical examination, vital signs were within normal limits. Body mass index was 22 kg/m². Deep tendon reflexes were decreased at the ankles but normal at the knees. Lower extremity muscle strength was normal. No abdominal or femoral bruit was present. No skin changes were noted in the lower extremities. Distal pulses were palpable bilaterally. The resting ankle-brachial index was 1.1 on both sides. How would you proceed with this case?

Case Review

This case scenario represents a patient with pseudoclaudication. This patient's normal ankle-brachial index bilaterally, normal distal pulses, lack of a bruit, normal skin findings, and clinical history all suggest a diagnosis other than peripheral arterial disease.

Case Discussion

Lumbar spinal stenosis can be described as an anatomic condition that involves narrowing of the central canal, lateral recess, and/or neural foramen.

Clinical Symptoms

Patients with pseudoclaudication (lumbar spinal stenosis) may report bilateral leg weakness associated with walking or with prolonged standing; symptoms are aggravated by prolonged standing and are relieved with bending at the waist. Nearly half of patients have absent deep tendon reflexes at the ankles, but reflexes at the knees and muscle strength are usually preserved.

Management

The American College of Physicians recommends that advanced imaging with MRI or CT should be reserved for patients with a suspected serious underlying condition or neurologic deficits or who are candidates for invasive interventions. In the absence of these indications, back imaging is not indicated. An MRI of the lumbar spine can be done in this patient to confirm the diagnosis. Conservative treatment is suggested for the patients with no fixed or progressive neurologic deficits. Conservative management includes physical therapy and/or oral pain medication. Surgical therapy is suggested for patients who do not have an adequate clinical response to conservative therapy and who are functionally disabled by their symptoms and for patients who have a progressive neurologic deficit.

Key Points

- Lumbar spinal stenosis is narrowing of the central canal, lateral recess, and/or neural foramen.
- Lumbar spinal stenosis may present as bilateral leg weakness associated with walking or with prolonged standing; symptoms are aggravated by prolonged standing and are relieved with bending at the waist.
- MRI or CT should be reserved for patients with a suspected serious underlying condition or neurologic deficits or for patients who are candidates for invasive interventions
- Conservative management includes physical therapy and/or oral pain medication. Surgical therapy is suggested for patients who do not have an adequate clinical response to conservative therapy and who are functionally disabled by their symptoms and for patients who have a progressive neurologic deficit.

CASE 3

Management of Upper Extremity Peripheral Arterial Disease (Subclavian Steal Syndrome)

A 70-year-old man presented to the emergency department with a 3-month history of left arm fatigue and dizziness. The patient reported that 2 days ago, he became dizzy while standing on a stool and looking for a toolbox in an overhead shelf with the left arm. He noticed that his symptoms improved after 2 minutes of rest. In addition, he stated that left arm activity reproduced his arm fatigue and discomfort, which was mainly in the forearm. He had a significant medical history of hyperlipidemia and hypertension. He denied any surgery in the past. He had a 50-pack-year smoking history, but he denied use of alcohol or recreational drugs. Home medications included lisinopril, amlodipine, and atorvastatin. On physical examination, he was afebrile, blood pressure was 115/65 mm Hg in the left arm and 147/89 mm Hg in the right arm, and pulse rate was 75 bpm. On auscultation, a bruit was heard over the left supraclavicular fossa. Right carotid upstroke was normal. The left radial pulse and left carotid pulse were faint, and the left radial pulse was slightly diminished. Cardiac examination was normal. Physical examination was otherwise unremarkable. How would you manage this case?

Case Review

This case scenario presents a patient with upper extremity peripheral arterial disease (PAD) and subclavian steal syndrome. The diagnosis was made based on the clinical presentation of left arm fatigue and dizziness with activity involving the left arm. The diagnosis was further supported by the physical examination findings such as significant difference in blood pressure between both arms, presence of bruit over the left supraclavicular fossa, and faint pulses over the left radial artery and left carotid artery. In addition, this patient had risk factors for PAD such as advanced age, smoking, hyperlipidemia, and hypertension.

Case Discussion

Upper extremity PAD is characterized by atherosclerotic narrowing of the arteries in the upper extremities. Most patients with upper extremity PAD have no symptoms, although patients may present with symptoms. In patients at risk for atherosclerotic cardiovascular disease, measurement of bilateral arm pressures is indicated in asymptomatic and symptomatic patients to assess for upper extremity PAD. A characteristic finding on physical examination is a difference in systolic blood pressures between the arms, typically >15 mm Hg.

Clinical Symptoms

Symptomatic patients with upper extremity PAD present with arm claudication, arm ischemia, or dizziness with arm activity (subclavian steal syndrome).

Management

The most appropriate next step in this patient suspected of having upper extremity PAD is CT angiography. Because this patient has arm claudication and a systolic blood pressure differential of 32 mm Hg between arms, imaging of the innominate and subclavian arteries with CT angiography is appropriate to confirm the diagnosis of upper extremity PAD and plan for intervention, such as revascularization. In addition, all patients should be managed with risk factor modifications, such as smoking cessation, high-intensity statins, and blood pressure control. Also, patients should be started on antiplatelet therapy, such as aspirin, to decrease the risk of myocardial infarctions, stroke, and peripheral arterial events. Furthermore, patients should be encouraged to enroll in the supervised exercise program, which can provide symptomatic relief. Patients should be started on cilostazol (a phosphodiesterase inhibitor with antiplatelet and vasodilator activity) for symptom relief. The decision for interventional therapy can be made based on the results of CT angiography.

Key Points

- Symptoms of upper extremity peripheral artery disease may include arm claudication, arm ischemia, or dizziness with arm activity.
- CT angiography is useful to confirm the diagnosis and plan for intervention.
- Smoking cessation is essential to reduce cardiovascular risk in patients with PAD. Antiplatelet monotherapy with aspirin is recommended for patients with PAD to reduce the risk for myocardial infarction, stroke, and peripheral arterial events. Supervised exercise training is the most effective treatment for improvement of functional status in patients with PAD. Cilostazol is recommended for patients with intermittent claudication.

CASE 4

Management of Acute Limb Ischemia

A 60-year-old man presented to the emergency department due to acute left lower leg pain that began 3 days ago. The pain was severe at rest, and he reported that his left foot was cold compared to the right foot. He was not able to do any activity due to the pain and felt the left leg was weak. He denied any fever, trauma, or neurologic deficits. His medical history was significant for intermittent claudication for the past 4 years, hypertension, hyperlipidemia, and type 2 diabetes mellitus. His surgical history was significant for left femoral-popliteal bypass graft surgery for life-limiting claudication 1.5 years ago. He was a former smoker who had quit smoking 5 years prior, and he denied alcohol use or recreational drug use. His medications were low-dose aspirin, ramipril, hydrochlorothiazide, rosuvastatin, and metformin. On physical examination, vital signs were within normal limits. The left foot was cold and pale compared to the right foot, sensations were intact, and muscle strength was normal. The pedal pulses were not palpable in the left leg. Arterial Doppler ultrasound signals were not detectable over the left dorsalis pedis and left posterior tibial arteries. He was started on intravenous anticoagulation with heparin. How would you manage this case further?

Case Review

This case scenario presents a patient with acute limb ischemia (ALI). The diagnosis of ALI was based on the history suggestive of acute pain in the left lower leg at rest; physical examination showing pallor, poikilothermia, and absence of pedal pulses in the left foot; and arterial Doppler ultrasound showing inability to detect signals over left dorsalis pedis and left posterior tibial artery. This patient has many risk factors for developing ALI, such as history of left femoral-popliteal bypass graft surgery for life-limiting claudication 1.5 years ago, former history of smoking, hypertension, hyperlipidemia, and diabetes mellitus type 2.

Case Discussion

ALI is defined by a sudden or rapid decrease in limb perfusion, often manifested as a new pulse deficit, rest pain, pallor, and/or paralysis. ALI is a medical emergency and a life-threatening manifestation of PAD. ALI is most commonly caused by acute thrombosis of a lower extremity artery, stent, or bypass graft. Other causes include thromboembolism, vessel dissection (usually occurring periprocedurally), or trauma.

Clinical Symptoms

Classically, patients present with at least 1 of the "6 Ps": paresthesia, pain, pallor, pulselessness, poikilothermia (coolness), and paralysis.

Management

Anticoagulation, typically with unfractionated heparin, should be initiated as soon as the diagnosis of ALI is suspected. The most appropriate next step in the management of this patient with ALI is urgent invasive angiography to determine the extent of disease and to plan treatment. Patients with ALI and a viable extremity are most commonly treated with surgical embolectomy or catheter-directed thrombolysis. This patient is demonstrating several classic signs of ALI, including pulselessness, pallor, and pain, and he is at heightened risk for ALI owing to his history of femoral-popliteal bypass graft surgery. The most appropriate next step is to perform invasive angiography to define the level of occlusion and to determine whether surgical embolectomy or catheter-directed thrombolysis is an option. Delay in treatment may lead to worsening limb perfusion, limb necrosis, or the need for lower extremity amputation. Noninvasive imaging studies, such as arterial duplex ultrasonography and CT angiography, may be useful to detect the level of stenosis and extent of disease, but these tests will substantially delay the treatment of ALI in this patient. This patient shows the signs of viability (intact sensation and muscle strength) and thus does not require immediate amputation. Emergent amputation is necessary in patients with ALI who have a nonviable extremity, such as gangrene or paralysis.

Key Points

- Patients present with at least 1 of the "6 Ps": paresthesia, pain, pallor, pulselessness, poikilothermia (coolness), and paralysis.
- Anticoagulation, typically with unfractionated heparin, should be initiated as soon as the diagnosis of ALI is suspected.
- In patients with ALI, invasive angiography should be performed immediately to define the anatomic level of occlusion and plan for revascularization.

CASE 5

Management of Critical Limb Ischemia

A 75-year-old man presented to the emergency department with a 4-week history of progressive right foot pain that occurred at rest. He also had calf muscle pain that worsened when he ambulated. His medical history was significant for type 2 diabetes mellitus, hypertension, and hyperlipidemia. The patient reported no significant surgeries in the past. He was a former smoker, who stopped smoking 5 years ago; he smoked 1 pack of cigarettes per day for 50 years before stopping. He denied use of alcohol or any other recreational drugs. Medications were low-dose aspirin, metformin, amlodipine, lisinopril, and rosuvastatin. On physical examination, vital signs were within normal limits. The right foot was cold. There was a shallow 3.5-cm × 2.8-cm ulceration on the medial aspect of the right first metatarsal. Pedal pulses were diminished on the left and absent on the right. Right foot sensations and muscle strength were intact. The ankle-brachial index (ABI) was calculated as 0.65 on the left and unobtainable on the right. How would you manage this case?

Case Review

This case scenario presents a patient with critical limb ischemia. The diagnosis was made by presence of rest pain and ulcer on clinical presentation, absent pulses on the left foot, and unobtainable ABI on the left side. In addition, this patient had risk factors for peripheral arterial disease (PAD) such as hypertension, diabetes mellitus, hyperlipidemia, and history of smoking for years.

Case Discussion

Critical limb ischemia is a severe form of PAD that is characterized by ischemic rest pain and ulceration. Clinical findings in a patient with critical limb ischemia include an ABI <0.40, a flat waveform on pulse volume recording, and low or absent pedal flow on duplex ultrasonography.

Management

The most appropriate next step in the management of this patient with critical limb ischemia is to perform invasive angiography of the affected limb with the intent to revascularize. Due to the high morbidity and mortality associated with critical limb ischemia, immediate invasive angiography with endovascular revascularization, without additional noninvasive imaging, is often the most effective strategy to preserve tissue viability. Imaging studies such as magnetic resonance angiography would result in treatment time delays in this patient with critical limb ischemia and a viable limb.

Endovascular or surgical revascularization procedures are effective in improving symptoms, increasing functional capacity, and improving wound healing in patients with intermittent claudication or critical limb ischemia. Referral for revascularization is indicated in patients with lifestyle-limiting claudication, rest pain, ulceration, or gangrene, especially if there has been an inadequate response to exercise training, cilostazol, and/or wound treatment. In patients with critical limb ischemia and a viable limb, angiography and revascularization are always preferred to primary major amputation of the lower extremity. Patients >65 years old who undergo major amputation have a 1-year mortality rate of nearly 50% and a 3-year mortality rate of >70%.

Key Points

- Critical limb ischemia is a severe form of PAD characterized by ischemic rest pain and ulceration.
- Clinical findings in a patient with critical limb ischemia include an ABI <0.40, a flat waveform on pulse volume recording, and low or absent pedal flow on duplex ultrasonography.
- In patients with critical limb ischemia, immediate invasive angiography with endovascular revascularization is often the most effective strategy to preserve tissue viability.

CASE 6

Management of Symptomatic Carotid Artery Disease

A 70-year-old woman presented to the emergency department due to a sudden episode of slurred speech and right-sided facial droop lasting approximately 2 minutes. The episode was preceded by flushing, dizziness, palpitations, and near-syncope. She had a medical history significant for diabetes mellitus, hypertension, coronary artery disease, hyperthyroidism, and severe peripheral vascular disease status post aortobifemoral bypass and right superficial femoral artery endarterectomy. Her social history included cigarettes smoking for the past 20 years. She denied any alcohol use or illicit drug use. On arrival, the patient was alert and oriented and in no acute distress. Vital signs were noted as blood pressure of 138/78 mm Hg in the right arm and 110/73 mm Hg in the left arm, heart rate of 83 bpm, respiratory rate of 18 breaths/min, and temperature of 98°F. Physical examination was completely noncontributory. Routine laboratory testing was normal. An ECG showed normal sinus rhythm. Initial head CT was normal. The patient was admitted to the telemetry floor. Carotid ultrasound indicated mild stenosis of the carotids bilaterally; anterograde right vertebral flow and reversed left vertebral flow suggested left proximal subclavian stenosis. Further neurovascular imaging was done. MRI of the head was normal, and magnetic resonance angiography showed a $3 \times 3 \times 6$ mm aneurysm arising from the left posterior communicating artery and a $2.3 \times 2 \times 3$ mm aneurysm on the left intracranial internal carotid artery (as shown in Figure 8.6.1). Decreased flow signal was found in the left vertebral artery. How would you manage this case?

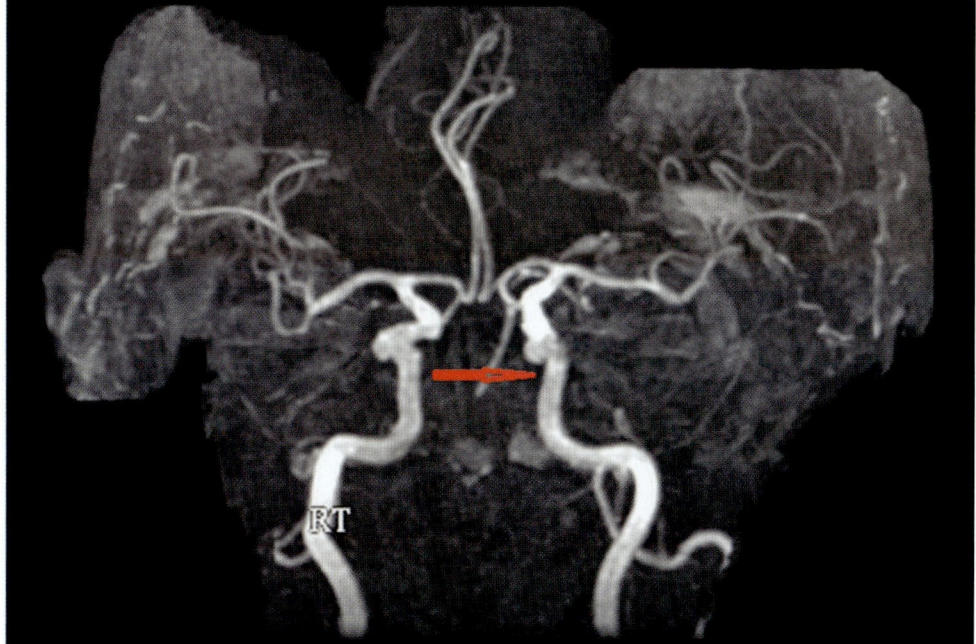

Figure 8.6.1 MRA showing a $3 \times 3 \times 6$ mm aneurysm arising from the left posterior communicating artery and a $2.3 \times 2 \times 3$ mm aneurysm on left intracranial internal carotid artery.

Case Review

The case presents a patient diagnosed with symptomatic moderate right carotid artery stenosis with mild left carotid stenosis, along with insidious multiple small intracranial aneurysms. In view of transient neurologic deficit with complete resolution of symptoms and no acute intracranial disease observed on neuroimaging, conservative medical management was adopted. This patient had a known history of vasculopathy with several prior interventions, for which risk factor modification was strongly encouraged, including smoking cessation, drug abstinence, and aggressive glycemic and blood pressure control.

Case Discussion

Carotid artery disease is associated with approximately 10% to 20% of all ischemic strokes. The carotid bifurcation is the most frequently affected location often extending to the proximal internal carotid artery. Progression of atheromatous plaque causes intraluminal narrowing and frequent ulceration, which may lead to transient ischemic attack or ischemic stroke from thrombosis, embolization, or hemodynamic instability. Identified histopathologic features of atheromatous plaques associated with elevated risk include the presence of inflammation, thrombus, lipid-rich necrotic core, and possibly intraplaque hemorrhage and thinning or rupture of the fibrous cap.

Clinical Symptoms

Sudden onset of focal neurologic symptoms in carotid artery distribution (ipsilateral to significant carotid atherosclerotic pathology) is seen.

Management

Treatment includes pharmacologic management (with statins, antiplatelet agents, and antihypertensive agents) and revascularization with carotid endarterectomy (CEA) and carotid artery stenting (CAS). Improvements in pharmacologic therapy have demonstrably reduced the risk of recurrent stroke; however, it continues to be a common dilemma in clinical practice to identify patients who can benefit from carotid intervention.

Current recommendations regarding benefits of intervention in symptomatic patients are based on the available data, which include 2 major trials comparing CEA versus medical therapy (North American Symptomatic Carotid Endarterectomy Trial [NASCET] and the European Carotid Surgery Trial [ECST]) performed between 1981 and 1996 and randomized trials (ICSS, SPACE, EVA-3S, and CREST) comparing CAS versus CEA. All recommendations regarding revascularization therapy are made with the provision that the perioperative risk of stroke and death for the surgeon, operator, or center is <6%.

Summarized recommendations based on the previously mentioned trials include the following:

- In symptomatic carotid stenosis of 70% to 99% in patients with a life expectancy of at least 5 years, CEA rather than medical management alone is recommended.
- CEA rather than CAS is recommended in symptomatic carotid stenosis of 70% to 99% with a life expectancy of at least 5 years when the following conditions are present:
  - A surgically accessible carotid lesion
  - Absence of clinically significant cardiac, pulmonary, or other disease that would greatly increase the risk of anesthesia and surgery
  - No prior ipsilateral endarterectomy

- Suggest CAS rather than CEA in carotid stenosis of 70% to 99%, in any of the following conditions:
  - A carotid lesion that is not suitable for surgical access
  - Radiation-induced stenosis
  - Clinically significant cardiac, pulmonary, or other disease that greatly increases the risk of anesthesia and surgery (however, it is not clear for this group whether revascularization outweighs medical management)
- The perioperative risk of stroke or death is approximately 2-fold higher with CAS compared with CEA for patients age 70 years and older with symptomatic carotid disease. Available evidence suggests the longer-term outcomes are similar for both CEA and CAS.
- Regarding sex, men with recently symptomatic carotid stenosis of 50% to 69% will benefit from CEA rather than medical therapy, but the opposite is true in women with carotid stenosis of 50% to 69%, who will benefit more from medical management rather than CEA.
- In symptomatic carotid stenosis <50%, medical management is recommended rather than CEA or CAS.
- CEA in a patient with carotid stenosis should be performed within 2 weeks rather than at a later time (but not in the first 48 hours due to evidence of associated increased risk) after onset of symptoms of a nondisabling stroke or transient ischemic attack (TIA).
- Patients with hemispheric TIA appear to have greater benefit from CEA than patients with transient retinal ischemia.

Key Points

- In symptomatic carotid stenosis of 70% to 99% in patients with a life expectancy of at least 5 years, CEA rather than medical management alone is recommended.
- Medical management is preferred over surgical intervention in patients with symptomatic carotid artery disease and high perioperative complication risk.

CASE 7

Management of Carotid Artery Dissection

A 29-year-old woman presented to the emergency department with a 2-day history of new-onset right-sided headache. The pain was located in the right temple and face and was not relieved by acetaminophen. She had no other symptoms and no significant medical history, except for heavy menstruation. She worked as a carpenter but never had any head trauma. She had menstruated heavily since puberty. The patient did not smoke or drink alcoholic beverages. On physical examination, temperature was 98.7°F, blood pressure was 105/70 mm Hg, pulse rate was 70 bpm, and respiration rate was 14 breaths/min; body mass index was 22.5 kg/m². The right pupil was 2 mm and the left pupil was 4 mm in size; both pupils were reactive to light. The patient was unable to close the left upper eyelid completely. There was no aphasia, nuchal rigidity, or hemiparesis. Results of laboratory studies were normal, including a total cholesterol level of 160 mg/dL and a high-density lipoprotein (HDL) cholesterol level of 60 mg/dL. Magnetic resonance angiography revealed >80% stenosis of the right internal carotid artery 4 cm above the bifurcation. An MRI of the brain was normal. How would you proceed further with this case?

Case Review

This case presents a patient with carotid artery dissection. Her clinical history and examination are most consistent with a right internal carotid artery dissection, as suggested by the headache and right partial Horner syndrome (presence of ptosis and miosis on the right). This diagnosis is further supported by arterial imaging, which shows stenosis in the right internal carotid artery that starts 4 cm above the bifurcation. An MRI is normal, without cerebral infarct.

Case Discussion

Dissection generally occurs when the structural integrity of the arterial wall is compromised, which allows blood to collect between layers as an intramural hematoma. Common causes include various degrees of trauma or spontaneous events, with underlying predispositions (connective tissue diseases) in some cases.

Clinical Symptoms

Patients with carotid artery dissection may present with stroke or transient ischemic attack (TIA); headache or neck pain at onset may suggest underlying dissection as a cause of stroke. The acute onset of Horner syndrome in association with neck pain and an ischemic stroke or TIA in the territory of the ipsilateral internal carotid artery are suggestive of spontaneous carotid artery dissection.

Diagnosis

The diagnosis of carotid artery dissection can be suspected by the clinical features and can be further supported by neuroimaging, such as MRI with magnetic resonance angiography (MRA) and CT with CT angiography (CTA). There is no need for conventional angiography if the diagnosis of cerebral or cervical artery dissection is clear using CTA or MRA.

Management

As per previous recommendations, patients with suspected internal carotid artery dissection are prescribed anticoagulation with warfarin to prevent an ischemic stroke from an embolism arising from the intimal tear. However, a recent study showed that antiplatelet agents were equivalent to warfarin in reducing stroke risk; this study also affirmed the overall low absolute risk of stroke in this disorder. Although the study was underpowered and did not establish superiority of one agent over the other, there are several reasons to recommend aspirin rather than warfarin in the patient in this case. Her employment as a carpenter places her at higher risk of trauma-associated bleeding, which could be excessive if she were taking warfarin; her heavy menses also argue against warfarin. This patient with probable carotid dissection has right internal carotid artery stenosis of a nonatherosclerotic origin as she has normal total and HDL cholesterol levels, is not a smoker, and is not hypertensive, indicating a low 10-year cardiovascular disease risk. Thus, a statin is unlikely to be necessary or useful.

Carotid artery stenting for carotid dissection has been studied in several case series in which patients have not responded to best medical therapy and have had >1 stroke. Carotid artery stenting poses a high risk in carotid dissection and is not indicated in this patient, who has not had a stroke and has no evidence of diminished cerebral blood flow. Novel anticoagulants (eg, rivaroxaban) have not been studied in carotid dissection, and their associated risks are likely to outweigh any potential clinical benefit in dissection.

Key Points

- Patients with carotid artery dissection may present with a stroke or TIA; headache or neck pain at onset may suggest underlying dissection as a cause of stroke. The acute onset of Horner syndrome in association with neck pain and an ischemic stroke or transient ischemic attack in the territory of the ipsilateral internal carotid artery are suggestive of spontaneous carotid artery dissection.
- Recent evidence showed that antiplatelet agents were equivalent to warfarin in reducing stroke risk.

CASE 8

Management of Giant Cell Arteritis

An 81-year-old man presented to the emergency department with acute-onset, left-sided vision loss. The patient reported transient visual loss in his left eye and later started having right-sided headaches along with difficulty in chewing food 3 weeks prior. The patient's past medical history included diabetes, hypertension, and peripheral vascular disease. He underwent a carotid duplex as an outpatient for the evaluation of his symptoms, which showed complete occlusion in the left internal carotid artery and stenosis of >70% in right internal carotid artery. The bilateral common and external carotid arteries were patent but diffusely atherosclerotic, with an estimated plaque burden of >40%. Based on the carotid duplex findings, he underwent a right carotid endarterectomy with no immediate complications. However, he continued to have persistent symptoms with progressive deterioration. He also noticed weight loss, anorexia, and morning stiffness in his shoulders.

On examination in the emergency department, his vital signs were within normal limits. The patient was cachectic and had right temporal and shoulder girdle tenderness. Pulses were diminished in all extremities. Bilateral carotid bruits were also appreciated. Visual acuity was noted to be 0/20 and 2/20 in the left and right eyes, respectively. Pupillary reflex was absent on the left side and sluggish on the right side. The rest of the neurologic system was grossly intact. Initial blood workup showed erythrocyte sedimentation rate (ESR) of 95 mm/h and C-reactive protein (CRP) of 10 mg/L. The complete blood cell count and metabolic profile were normal. The patient was examined by an ophthalmologist who detected ischemic optic changes. He was transferred to the telemetry floor. How would you manage this case further?

Case Review

This case scenario presents a patient with suspected giant cell arteritis (GCA), which can mimic stroke or carotid artery disease. In this patient, GCA was suspected by the clinical symptoms of acute vision loss on the left side, blurry vision on the right side, jaw claudication, and right-sided headache. The clinical symptoms were further supported by findings of the physical examination such as right temporal tenderness and bilateral carotid bruits. Furthermore, the patient was examined by an ophthalmologist as an outpatient and was found to have ischemic optic changes highly suggestive of GCA. Finally, the lab findings of elevated ESR and CRP were supportive for suspected GCA.

Case Discussion

GCA is characterized by granulomatous inflammation of affected vessels with infiltration of lymphocytes, macrophages, and multinucleated giant cells. Involved vessels include the aorta, its major branches off the arch, and secondary branch vessels, including the external carotid, subclavian, axillary, temporal, ophthalmic, ciliary, occipital, and vertebral arteries. The level of vessel involved dictates the clinical symptoms.

Clinical Symptoms

Symptoms of GCA generally include headache, scalp pain, and temporal artery tenderness. Symptoms are frequently unilateral but can be bilateral. Aching and fatigue with chewing (jaw claudication) indicate ischemia of the muscles of mastication. Fever, fatigue, and weight loss may be present. The most feared complication is ischemic optic neuropathy, which can cause amaurosis fugax and blindness. Physical examination may reveal scalp or temporal artery tenderness and induration, reduced pulses and bruits, or aortic regurgitation and heart failure. Up to 50% of patients with GCA have polymyalgia rheumatica (PMR), which may occur before, concurrent with, or following diagnosis of GCA.

Diagnosis

Laboratory findings may include elevated ESR and/or CRP, but some patients have normal values. GCA is suspected based on the clinical presentation and is confirmed by temporal artery biopsy and/or imaging of the great vessels. New or atypical headache, jaw claudication, or visual changes in a patient over the age of 50 years, especially with concurrent PMR, should raise suspicion. Temporal artery biopsy is diagnostic, but false-negative results are common; bilateral temporal artery biopsy can increase the yield.

Management

Suspected GCA must be treated immediately with steroids to prevent visual loss. Prednisone, 1 mg/kg/d, is recommended. Intravenous pulse methylprednisolone for 3 days is used for acute visual loss, but established blindness is usually irreversible. The efficacy of the treatment can be monitored by symptoms and inflammatory markers because they usually respond rapidly to glucocorticoids; lack of response should prompt reconsideration of the diagnosis. High-dose prednisone is maintained for 2 to 4 weeks; after symptoms resolve and inflammatory markers normalize, prednisone is tapered by 10% to 20% every 2 weeks. Once a dose of 10 mg/d is reached, the taper is slowed to 1 mg per month. While on the treatment, patient should be monitored for recurrence of the symptoms, and ESR and CRP should be monitored every month. Glucocorticoid-sparing immunosuppressives such as methotrexate are sometimes used, although little data support their efficacy. The interleukin-6 inhibitor tocilizumab was recently approved by the US Food and Drug Administration for treatment of GCA.

Key Points

- Symptoms of GCA generally include headache, scalp pain, visual changes, and temporal artery tenderness. Jaw claudication, fever, weight loss, or fatigue may be present.
- Laboratory findings may include elevated ESR and/or CRP, but some patients have normal values.

- Suspected GCA must be treated immediately with steroids to prevent visual loss. Prednisone 1 mg/kg/d is recommended. Intravenous pulse methylprednisolone for 3 days is used for acute visual loss, but established blindness is usually irreversible.

CASE 9

Management of Asymptomatic Carotid Artery Stenosis

A 70-year-old man was sent from the clinic to the emergency department for a blood pressure (BP) of 190/95 mm Hg. The patient had been complaining of headache, palpitations, and dizziness since the morning. The patient reported that his BP at home was also high that morning and he had not taken any medications for the past 2 days because he had run out of medication. The patient had a medical history of hypertension. His home medications for hypertension included amlodipine and lisinopril. Other medications included aspirin and atorvastatin. He did not have any past surgical history. He was a former smoker and stopped smoking 10 years ago; he denied use of alcohol or recreational drugs. Review of systems was otherwise unremarkable. On physical examination, his BP was elevated, and carotid bruits were present on both sides; otherwise, the physical examination was unremarkable. Laboratory results showed complete blood count and metabolic profile within normal range. In the emergency department, the patient's BP was controlled using labetalol, and the symptoms resolved. The patient was admitted to the telemetry floor for monitoring. CT of the head was normal. Carotid duplex was done and showed 50% stenosis in the right internal carotid artery and 40% stenosis in the left internal carotid artery. The patient's BP was well controlled, and he was resumed on his home medications. How would you manage carotid artery stenosis in this patient?

Case Review

This case scenario presents a patient with asymptomatic carotid artery stenosis. The patient presented with the symptoms of headache, palpitations, and intermittent dizziness, which resolved after controlling the high BP. The patient was found to have bilateral carotid artery stenosis by presence of carotid bruits on both sides and per findings of the carotid duplex. However, the patient had no symptoms related to carotid artery stenosis.

Case Discussion

Asymptomatic carotid atherosclerotic disease refers to atherosclerotic narrowing of the extracranial carotid artery without a history of stroke or transient ischemic attack. Carotid stenosis does not cause vertigo, lightheadedness, or syncope. Therefore, these symptoms should not be considered as symptomatic carotid artery disease. Patients with asymptomatic carotid atherosclerotic disease are at risk of developing stroke, myocardial ischemia, and vascular death. Thus, intensive medical management of asymptomatic carotid artery atherosclerotic disease is important.

Management

The management of asymptomatic carotid atherosclerotic disease is controversial. Management of carotid artery disease includes pharmacologic management, surgical intervention, and lifestyle modifications. Medical management mainly includes use of statins and antiplatelet agents, treatment of hypertension and diabetes, and healthy lifestyle changes and has narrowed the gap between medical and surgical treatment of carotid disease for reducing the risk of stroke and other cardiovascular disease. Surgical intervention is reserved for symptomatic cases. In addition to medical and surgical management, lifestyle modifications play an important role.

Key Points

- Asymptomatic carotid atherosclerotic disease is atherosclerotic narrowing of the extracranial carotid artery without a history of stroke or transient ischemic attack.
- Medical management mainly includes use of statins and antiplatelet agents, treatment of hypertension and diabetes, and healthy lifestyle changes and has narrowed the gap between medical and surgical treatment of carotid disease for reducing the risk of stroke and other cardiovascular disease.

CASE 10

Management of Carotid Artery Disease Risk Factors

A 45-year-old man presented to emergency department with complaints of dizziness and frequent headaches. These symptoms occurred intermittently over the past few weeks and were not associated with blurry vision, weakness, numbness, or loss of consciousness. He had not sought medical care until his symptoms eventually made him unable to work in the field. However, no symptoms of coronary artery disease were present. He had a significant medical history of familial hypercholesterolemia but was not on any lipid-lowering medications at the time of presentation. He had a family history of coronary artery disease in his father. The patient had no other cardiovascular risk factors such as smoking, high blood pressure, or diabetes mellitus and was physically active. On physical examination, neck auscultation revealed a bruit in the neck, radiating to the skull. In addition, he had xanthomas on the elbows, soles of the feet, and Achilles tendons. ECG, chest radiography, stress testing, telemetry monitoring, and echocardiography revealed no abnormalities. The patient's low- and high-density lipoprotein cholesterol levels were 550 and 50 mg/dL, respectively. Ultrasonography of the carotid arteries showed severe stenosis in the left internal carotid artery (LICA), with stenosis estimated between 70% and 90%, and moderate stenosis in the right internal carotid artery (RICA), estimated between 40% and 50%. Ultrasonography also showed the presence of plaques in the anterior and posterior walls of the internal carotid artery and common carotid artery, which were characterized as bulky plates extending to the middle third of the internal coronary arteries and as predominantly echogenic and hyperechoic, with <50% of the area being echolucent with uneven surfaces. How would you manage this case?

Case Review

In this case, the risk factor for carotid artery disease was familial hypercholesterolemia. The diagnosis was based on presence of bruits on neck auscultation and carotid duplex ultrasound findings. Carotid ultrasound showed severe stenosis (70% to 90%) in the LICA and moderate stenosis (40% to 50%) in the RICA. In addition, carotid duplex ultrasound showed the presence of plaques in the anterior and posterior walls of the internal carotid artery and common carotid artery. This patient does not qualify for surgical intervention.

Case Discussion

Familial hypercholesterolemia (FH) is an autosomal dominant condition associated with coronary, carotid, and peripheral artery disease. It has been reported that carotid artery disease in FH occurs earlier than coronary artery disease. Carotid artery disease occurs when fatty deposits (plaques) clog the blood vessels that deliver blood to the brain and head (carotid arteries). Plaque buildup can lead to narrowing or blockage in the carotid artery, which, when significant, can put an individual at increased risk for stroke.

Other risk factors for carotid artery disease include hypertension, diabetes mellitus, tobacco smoking, obesity, dyslipidemia, advanced age, atrial fibrillation, sleep apnea, lack of exercise, and family history.

Clinical Symptoms

Carotid artery disease usually presents with no early signs or symptoms, and thus, the condition goes unnoticed. However, in some patients with late stages, it may present as either transient ischemic attack (TIA) or stroke. The signs and symptoms suggestive of TIA or stroke include sudden onset of numbness or weakness in the face or limbs, often on only one side of the body, trouble speaking and understanding, trouble seeing in 1 or both eyes, dizziness or loss of balance, and severe headache with no known cause.

Diagnosis

The presence of carotid bruits on neck auscultation is suggestive of carotid artery stenosis. Such physical examination findings need to be investigated further using noninvasive testing to confirm the diagnosis of carotid artery disease. Commonly used noninvasive tests include carotid duplex ultrasound, CT angiogram, magnetic resonance angiogram, and carotid angiography. Among these noninvasive testing modalities, carotid duplex ultrasound is the most commonly used test because of its wide availability, low cost, and low risk. In some cases, CT of the brain would be beneficial when it is suspected that stroke or TIA has already occurred.

Management

Management of carotid artery disease includes medical management, surgical intervention, and lifestyle modifications. Lipid-lowering therapy is the cornerstone of management. All patients with carotid artery disease should be placed on telemetry monitoring to detect any cardiac arrhythmias, especially atrial fibrillation. In addition, such patients need to be placed on antiplatelets because they are at high risk of developing stroke or other cardiovascular complications. As surgical interventions, carotid endarterectomy (CEA) and carotid angioplasty and stenting (CAS) have been proven to be beneficial for symptomatic patients with a 50% or greater carotid stenosis (blockage) and for asymptomatic patients with a 60% or greater carotid stenosis. When the degree of stenosis is <50%, there is no indication for carotid revascularization by either CEA or CAS. In addition to medical and surgical management, lifestyle modifications play an important role. Lifestyle modifications include strategies to reduce risk factors such as quitting smoking, controlling high blood pressure or glucose, following a low-cholesterol diet, losing weight, limiting alcohol intake, and exercising regularly.

Key Points

- Risk factors for carotid artery disease include hypertension, diabetes mellitus, tobacco smoking, obesity, dyslipidemia, advanced age, atrial fibrillation, sleep apnea, lack of exercise, and family history.
- The presence of carotid bruits on neck auscultation is suggestive of carotid artery stenosis.
- Management of carotid artery disease includes medical management (antiplatelet therapy to prevent stroke), surgical interventions (CEA or CAS), and lifestyle modifications.

9

10 Real Cases on Electrolyte Management and Miscellaneous Cases on Telemetry

Niel Shah • Nisha Ali • Jeirym Miranda • Muhammad Saad

CASE 1

Management of Hypernatremia

A 68-year-old male nursing home resident was brought to the emergency department by emergency medical services for altered mental status since early morning. As per nursing home staff, the patient had been experiencing poor oral intake and had been noted to be withdrawn from social activities over the past few days. Review of system was negative for nausea, vomiting, diarrhea, or fever. His medical history included hypertension, hyperlipidemia, osteoarthritis, and dementia. His medications included amlodipine, simvastatin, and multivitamins. Physical examination showed stable vital signs. However, the patient was cachectic, had dry mucous membranes, was alert and awake, and was able to follow commands but was confused. The rest of the examination was completely unremarkable. Significant laboratory data showed sodium of 167 mmol/L, chloride of 125 mmol/L, potassium of 4.0 mmol/L, and creatinine of 1.8 mg/dL (137.25 μmol/L). His cell count was normal. CT of the head showed no acute infarct, mass, or hemorrhages as well as no chronic microvascular changes. He was started on intravenous fluid and was transferred to the telemetry unit for electrolyte monitoring. How would you manage this case?

Case Review

The case presents a common scenario where an elderly nursing home resident with poor oral intake is admitted with acute altered level of consciousness due to poor eating and has responded to fluids. Hypernatremia should be managed cautiously in this case, and frequent monitoring of sodium level should be performed. Rapid correction can lead to central pontine myelinolysis.

Case Discussion

Hypernatremia is defined as a serum sodium concentration >145 mmol/L. It reflects a total body water deficit relative to total body sodium content caused by decreased water intake compared to water losses. The risk factors for development of hypernatremia include advanced age, mental or physical impairment, diuretic therapy, uncontrolled diabetes (solute diuresis), underlying polyuria disorders, nursing home resident, inadequate nursing care, and hospitalization.

Classification of Hypernatremia. Importantly, extracellular fluid (ECF) volume status should be assessed because it shows total body sodium content.

- Hypovolemic hypernatremia: Decreased total body water (TBW) and sodium with a relatively greater decrease in TBW. It includes gastrointestinal losses (diarrhea, vomiting), skin losses (burns or excessive sweating), and renal loss (intrinsic renal disease, osmotic [glucose, urea, mannitol] and loop diuretics).
- Euvolemic hypernatremia: Decreased TBW with near-normal total body sodium. It includes extrarenal losses from the respiratory tract (tachypnea) or skin (excessive sweating or fever), renal losses (central diabetes insipidus or nephrogenic diabetes insipidus), and other causes (inability to access water, primary hypodipsia, reset osmostat).
- Hypervolemic hypernatremia: Increased sodium with normal or increased TBW. It includes hypertonic fluid administration (hypertonic saline, sodium bicarbonate, total parenteral nutrition) and mineralocorticoid excess (adrenal tumors, congenital adrenal hyperplasia).

Clinical Symptoms

Thirst is a major symptom with dehydration or clinical signs of volume depletion. Other symptoms include neurologic symptoms such as generalized weakness, confusion, neuromuscular excitability, hyperreflexia, seizures, and coma.

Management

The approach to therapy is based on:

- Estimating water deficit = Current TBW × [(Serum [Na]/140) − 1]
- Designing the fluid repletion regimen:
  - Acute: Hourly infusion rate (mL/h) > Water deficit in mL ÷ 24 hours
  - Chronic: Desired water replacement in the first day in mL = 3 mL/kg body weight × 10 hourly infusion rate (mL/h) = Desired water replacement in the first day in mL ÷ 24 hours
- Determining the appropriate rate of correction (rapid lowering of sodium concentration can lead to cerebral edema in chronic hypernatremia, and untreated acute hypernatremia can cause permanent neurologic injury):
  - Acute hypernatremia (<48 hours, uncommon; seen in patients with use of salt tablets, uncontrolled diabetes insipidus, severe hyperglycemia):
    - Goal is to lower the serum sodium by 1 to 2 mmol/L per hour and to achieve normonatremia in <24 hours.
    - Dextrose 5% in water intravenously (IV) at a rate of 3 to 6 mL/kg/h.

- Reduce to 1 mL/kg/h once sodium concentration has reached 145 mmol/L and continue until normonatremia (140 mmol/L) is restored.
  - Monitor serum sodium and blood glucose every 2 to 3 hours until sodium is <145 mmol/L.
- Chronic hypernatremia (>48 hours; nearly all patients with hypernatremia):
  - Goal is to lower the serum sodium by a maximum of 10 mmol/L in a 24-hour period.
  - Dextrose 5% in water IV at a rate of approximately 1.35 mL/h × patient's weight in kilograms, or approximately 70 mL/h in a 50-kg patient and 100 mL/h in a 70-kg patient.
- While correcting hypernatremia, simultaneously monitor fluid status and urine output, repeat weight (initially every 6 hours, especially for infants or those with severe hypernatremia), monitor other electrolytes and blood sugar, measure ongoing losses (ie, vomiting or diarrhea, excluding urine) and replace milliliter for milliliter with normal saline, and perform careful neurologic monitoring.
- Patients with central diabetes insipidus will also require desmopressin therapy.

Key Points

- Hypernatremia requires assessment of volume status and fluid deficit.
- Acute hyponatremia should be treated with caution.

CASE 2

Management of Hyponatremia

A 47-year-old woman was brought to the hospital by a friend for generalized fatigue, myalgia, and lethargy after running a marathon. As per the patient, she was in her usual state of health that morning prior to the marathon and was a healthy and physically active woman. She denied skipping a meal, nausea, vomiting, or neurologic deficit. She had no significant medical comorbidities and only took over-the-counter multivitamins. The patient denied any alcohol, tobacco, or illicit drug use. No significant family history was noted. In the emergency department, her vitals were noted as blood pressure of 120/83 mm Hg, heart rate of 103 bpm, respiratory rate of 20 breaths/min, and temperature of 98.6°F. Her physical examination, including a complete neurologic examination, was unremarkable. Chest x-ray was normal. Initial laboratory data showed hemoglobin of 11 g/dL, blood urea nitrogen of 20 mg/dL, creatinine of 0.9 mg/dL, sodium of 120 mmol/L (120 mEq/L), chloride of 80 mmol/L (80 mEq/L), potassium of 3.9 mmol/L (3.9 mEq/L), and creatinine kinase of 300 mg/dL. Urine drug screen was negative, and urine specific gravity was 1.10. She was started on normal saline bolus and was transferred to the telemetry floor. How would you manage this case?

Case Review

This case presents a healthy adult athlete with acute asymptomatic hyponatremia. Further assessment of volume status and urine and serum osmolarity should be performed, and careful correction of sodium should be initiated. Sodium levels should be monitored frequently, and the correction should not exceed 4 to 6 mmol/L in the first 24 hours. The cause of her hyponatremia was most likely water intoxication in the setting of marathon and free water intake. Hypertonic saline can be used in acute symptomatic hyponatremia.

Case Discussion

Hyponatremia is defined as serum sodium <135 mmol/L, representing a relative excess of water in relation to sodium. Volume assessment along with serum and urine osmolarity should be performed to identify the etiology. Common causes include heart failure, renal failure, hypothyroidism, syndrome of inappropriate antidiuretic hormone secretion (SIADH), psychogenic polydipsia, diuretic use, hypercortisolism, and poor oral intake.

It can be either acute or chronic (development of hyponatremia over ≥48 hours).

Clinical Symptoms

Symptoms include nausea, vomiting, dizziness, headache, muscle cramps, fatigue, gait disturbances, forgetfulness, confusion and lethargy, obtundation, coma, seizures, and respiratory arrest.

Management

The treatment depends on the duration of the hyponatremia (acute or chronic). Patients with acute symptomatic hyponatremia should receive management in hospital settings for frequent assessments of neurologic status, accurate serum sodium concentration, and urine output.

In hospitalized patients, the treatment goal is to prevent further decrease in the serum sodium concentration, to relieve symptoms of hyponatremia, to decrease intracerebral pressure in those at risk for development of brain herniation, and to avoid excessive correction of hyponatremia in patients at risk for osmotic demyelination syndrome (ODS).

The goal of initial therapy is to raise the serum sodium concentration by 4 to 6 mmol/L in a 24-hour period.

Acute hyponatremia can be corrected by using a bolus of 3% saline (ie, hypertonic saline) to prevent a decrease in the serum sodium.

Chronic hyponatremia can be corrected by identification of the offending cause and its reversal such as medication. In symptomatic cases, 3% saline can be used with simultaneous use of desmopressin to prevent rapid correction among those who are at high risk of developing ODS.

Hypertonic saline should be discontinued once the daily correction goal of 4 to 6 mmol/L has been achieved and can be resumed as needed to preserve the desired increase in serum sodium for the day if it begins to fall again.

In addition to the specific therapies that are aimed at correcting the hyponatremia, therapy should also be directed at the underlying disease.

Fluid restriction below the level of urine output is indicated in edematous states such as heart failure, cirrhosis, advanced renal impairment, SIADH, and primary polydipsia.

Other therapies may include oral salt tablets, loop diuretics, potassium supplementation, urea, or vasopressin receptor antagonists depending on the etiology of hyponatremia.

Key Points

- Symptomatic hyponatremia should be treated with hypertonic saline and slow correction of sodium levels.
- Identification of etiology and reversal of offending agents are key in management.

CASE 3

Management of Hyperkalemia

A 58-year-old man presented to the emergency department (ED) with complaints of malaise and weakness since the morning. He reported using ibuprofen for knee pain for the past 2 days and had missed his last 2 hemodialysis sessions because he was not feeling good. His medical history included hypertension, end-stage renal disease (on hemodialysis), diabetes mellitus, and osteoarthritis of the knees. Medications included aspirin, atorvastatin, losartan, sevelamer, and carvedilol. In the ED, he was vitally stable. Physical examination revealed bibasilar crackles and pitting edema of the bilateral lower extremities. Laboratory results showed serum potassium of 7.9 mmol/L and creatinine of 11 mg/dL. His ECG (shown in the Figure 9.3.1) showed normal sinus rhythm with tall T waves in anterior precordial leads. The patient received calcium chloride, insulin, and dextrose. Emergent hemodialysis was planned. How would you manage this case?

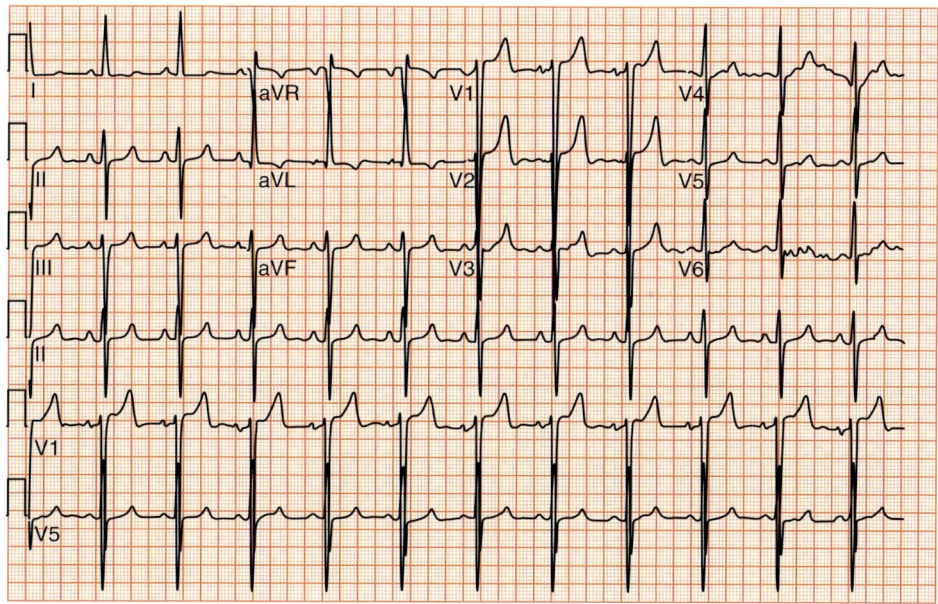

Figure 9.3.1 ECG showing normal sinus rhythm with tall T waves in anterior precordial leads.

Case Review

This case describes the management of hyperkalemia. Missed hemodialysis can lead to hyperkalemia, which can present as malaise, weakness, and bradycardia. Intravenous calcium chloride, potassium-binding resins, and insulin therapy can be used to treat hyperkalemia. Any offending medication should be stopped. If unresponsive to medical therapy, emergent hemodialysis should be performed.

Case Discussion

Potassium level >5.5 mmol/L is considered hyperkalemia. The severity is classified as follows: mild, 5.5 to 5.9 mmol/L; moderate, 6.0 to 6.4 mmol/L; and severe, >6.5 mmol/L. It is caused by impaired urinary potassium excretion due to acute or chronic kidney disease or disorders or drugs that inhibit the renin-angiotensin-aldosterone system.

Common causes include kidney failure, hypoaldosteronism, and rhabdomyolysis. Medications that cause high blood potassium include spironolactone, nonsteroidal anti-inflammatory drugs, and angiotensin-converting enzyme inhibitors. Pseudo-hyperkalemia, due to breakdown of cells during or after taking the blood sample, should be ruled out.

Diagnosis is usually made based on laboratory and ECG finding (prolongation of the PR interval, development of peaked T waves, widening of the QRS complex, and ECG complex that evolved to a sinusoidal shape).

Clinical Symptoms

Symptoms include malaise, weakness, paralysis, arrhythmias, and cardiac arrest.

Management

Patients with signs and symptoms of hyperkalemia or ECG changes require prompt therapy with intravenous calcium to stabilize cardiac myocyte membrane potential. Intravenous insulin (typically given with dextrose) can be used to drive extracellular potassium into the cells. To remove potassium from the body, gastrointestinal cation exchanger and/or dialysis can be used.

Treatment of reversible causes of hyperkalemia, such as discontinuing offending drugs, should be the cornerstone of management.

Key Points

- Hyperkalemia should be treated promptly to prevent life-threatening arrhythmias and sudden cardiac death.
- Hyperkalemia emergencies should be treated with insulin, dextrose, calcium chloride, or gluconate plus cation gastrointestinal exchangers and hemodialysis.

CASE 4

Management of Hypokalemia

A 45-year-old man presented to the emergency department with complaints of diarrhea and generalized weakness for the past 2 days. The symptoms were associated with poor appetite. He denied nausea, vomiting, dizziness, and weight loss. His medical history included newly diagnosed hypertension, and his medications included hydrochlorothiazide. He denied any family history of malignancy. On physical examination, he was vitally stable. Cardiac, pulmonary, and neurologic examinations revealed no abnormalities. Laboratory data revealed serum sodium of 132 mmol/L and potassium of 2.7 mmol/L. His kidney function was normal. ECG showed normal sinus rhythm with decrease in amplitude of T wave and appearance of U wave. The patient was started on intravenous fluids and intravenous potassium chloride replacement and was transferred to the telemetry floor for further monitoring. What is the cause of this patient's hypokalemia?

Case Review

This case describes the causes and management of hypokalemia. In this particular scenario, hypokalemia is caused by gastrointestinal loss due to diarrhea with concomitant use of a diuretic (hydrochlorothiazide). The ECG changes are characteristic for hypokalemia, and potassium replacement and hydration should be initiated.

Case Discussion

Serum potassium level <3.5 mmol/L is defined as hypokalemia. A potassium level <2.5 mmol/L is classified as severe hypokalemia. The most common causes of hypokalemia are gastrointestinal or urinary losses due to vomiting, diarrhea, or diuretic therapy. It may also result from the transient entry of potassium into cells, known as redistributive hypokalemia.

Urine potassium loss >20 mmol per 24 hours suggests excessive urinary loss, whereas level <20 mmol per 24 hours suggests cellular shift or extrarenal loss.

Hypokalemia is diagnosed by laboratory testing and ECG findings (QRS prolongation, ST-segment and T-wave depression, and U-wave formation).

Clinical Symptoms

Symptoms include weakness, fatigue, myalgia, leg cramps, constipation, flaccid paralysis, hyporeflexia, arrhythmias, and cardiac arrest.

Management

Treatment includes identification of underlying conditions such as diarrhea or removing offending medication. Mild hypokalemia (>3.0 mmol/L) may be treated by increased intake of potassium-containing foods or by oral potassium chloride supplements. Patients with severe hypokalemia (<3.0 mmol/L) or those with arrythmias or symptomatic hypokalemia may require intravenous supplementation. When replacing potassium intravenously using high concentrations, infusion by a central line is encouraged to avoid phlebitis or caustic effects at the site of infusion. Magnesium depletion should be assessed and corrected in refractory hypokalemia. Resistant hypokalemia is treated with a potassium-sparing diuretic such as amiloride, triamterene, spironolactone, or eplerenone. Patients with primary hyperaldosteronism also present with hypokalemia. Spironolactone or eplerenone can be used in those cases.

Key Points

- Prompt correction of hypokalemia is required to prevent life-threatening arrhythmias and sudden cardiac death.
- Oral supplementation is always preferred over the intravenous route if not contraindicated.

CASE 5

Management of Hypomagnesemia

A 61-year-old woman came to the emergency department (ED) with a complaint of shortness of breath that started 2 days ago that progressively worsened to the point that she could not walk or perform activities. She used 3 pillows to sleep and had to wake up in the night to breathe. She denied chest pain, cough, sick contact, headache, and fatigue. Her medical history was significant for heart failure with reduced ejection fraction (nonischemic cardiomyopathy), hypertension, and hyperlipidemia. She had been taking all her medications daily but missed a few doses of furosemide because she ran out of the prescriptions. Her home medications included furosemide, lisinopril, carvedilol, and atorvastatin. Her social history and family history were not significant. In the ED, her vital signs were noted as temperature of 98.6°F, heart rate of 85 bpm, blood pressure of 125/85 mm Hg, and oxygen saturation of 98% on 2-L nasal cannula. On physical examination, she had elevated jugular venous distention, S_3 heart sound, and rales in two-thirds of the lung field bilaterally. She also had bilateral pitting edema up to the shin. The rest of the physical examination was completely unremarkable. ECG showed normal sinus rhythm and left ventricular hypertrophy. The chest x-ray showed interstitial edema bilaterally. Laboratory testing showed elevated pro-B-type natriuretic peptide with electrolyte levels as follows: potassium of 4 mmol/L, creatinine of 0.8 mg/dL, and magnesium of 1.4 mmol/L. She was given 1 dose of intravenous furosemide in the ED and was transferred to the telemetry floor for heart failure management. On the floor, her symptoms started improving with furosemide, but she was noticed to have a magnesium level of 0.8 mmol/L on subsequent lab testing. Potassium and creatinine levels remained normal. How would you manage low magnesium in this patient?

Case Review

This case highlights the management of electrolytes in a heart failure patient. Potassium and magnesium should be adequately managed with furosemide therapy because they can worsen the symptoms. Oral or intravenous magnesium should be used to replenish the losses, and diuretic therapy can be continued simultaneously. Potassium-sparing diuretics can be used, and dietary magnesium content should be increased. Persistently low magnesium can lead to QT prolongation and fatal arrhythmias.

Case Discussion

Hypomagnesemia is commonly associated with hypokalemia and hypocalcemia. It can be found in patients with poor intake and malnourished individuals. A serum level of <1.8 mmol/L is used to diagnose hypomagnesemia, and a level <1.4 mmol/L is considered severe hypomagnesemia. The deficiency should also be suspected in cases with refractory hypokalemia and hypocalcemia. The most common etiologies include chronic alcoholism, chronic diarrhea, and medications such as diuretics, cisplatin, proton pump inhibitors, and amphotericin.

Clinical Symptoms

Symptoms include fatigue, lethargy, muscle cramps, tremors, and hyperreflexia.

Management

Oral supplements are usually required to treat hypomagnesemia, with intravenous formulations reserved for patients with intolerance to oral therapy or patients with severe symptoms. In severe symptomatic cases (eg, seizures), 2 to 4 g of intravenous magnesium sulfate can be used over 5 to 10 minutes; the dose can be repeated to total of 10 g over 6 hours. In less severe cases, 50 mmol of magnesium sulfate may be given intravenously in

5% dextrose in water over a 24-hour period. Lower concentrations should be used in acute kidney injury. Patients should be monitored for fatal arrhythmias, and magnesium levels should be checked frequently. Correction of hypokalemia and hypocalcemia should also be continued.

In diuretic-associated hypomagnesemia, the addition of a potassium-sparing diuretic (amiloride or triamterene) can provide benefit. A diet rich in magnesium such as dairy products, seafood, and cereals should be emphasized. In refractory cases, oral magnesium supplements can be used to reach the magnesium goal.

Key Points
- Hypomagnesemia is diagnosed with serum levels <1.8 mmol/L.
- Etiology includes chronic alcoholism, diarrhea, and medications such as diuretics.
- Oral supplements should be used in asymptomatic cases, with intravenous magnesium reserved for symptomatic cases.
- Hypokalemia and hypocalcemia should be corrected.

CASE 6

Perioperative Medication Management

A 65-year-old man presented to the hospital after falling at home. He stated that he was walking on an uneven surface and twisted his leg. He denied dizziness, headache, loss of consciousness, and palpitations. His medical history included heart failure with reduced ejection fraction (ejection fraction, 38%), coronary artery disease, hypertension, and hyperlipidemia. His home medications included aspirin, atorvastatin, carvedilol, and lisinopril. In the emergency department, the vital signs were stable. Physical examination showed an asymmetric leg. Cardiovascular examination was unremarkable. X-ray showed displaced fracture of the left femur head. The orthopedics team scheduled the patient for left side total hip replacement. His ECG showed normal sinus rhythm and Q waves in leads II, III, and aVF. Initial laboratory testing was unremarkable. He was admitted to the telemetry floor. How would you manage this patient's medications before surgery?

Case Review

This case describes the management of perioperative medications for congestive heart failure (CHF) and coronary artery disease (CAD) patients. In certain circumstances, a telemetry resident or physician is required to provide preoperative clearance. For elective surgery, preoperative care should be optimized to reduce the risk of a major adverse cardiovascular event (MACE). Heart failure medications should be optimized and continued perioperatively. The fact that this patient has CHF and CAD should not delay the surgery if he does not have active angina or heart failure symptoms.

Case Discussion

Patients planned for emergent surgery should not be delayed for surgery due to cardiac testing, whereas surgery should not be performed in patients with ongoing ischemia. Asymptomatic patients with no cardiovascular risk factors should proceed with surgery. In patients with cardiovascular risk factors, risk of MACE can be estimated by using the Revised Cardiac Risk Index (RCRI) calculator. The RCRI includes high-risk surgery, ischemic heart disease, heart failure, chronic kidney disease, and diabetes mellitus requiring insulin. In low-risk surgeries such as cataract extraction and inguinal hernia repair, cardiac testing should not be performed even with elevated RCRI score. In patients with elevated MACE risk (>1%), functional capacity should be assessed using metabolic equivalents (METs). An exercise capacity >4 METs is considered good, and no cardiac testing is required. Exercise testing can be performed to further assess poor exercise capacity if it will change the management prior to surgery. ECG can be performed for asymptomatic patients with unknown CAD. It is reasonable to obtain ECG within 3 months of surgery for any patient with known CAD, arrhythmia, or cerebrovascular accident. Echocardiogram can be considered if symptoms are suggestive of heart failure or valvular heart disease or worsening of condition.

β-Blockers. β-Blockers reduce ischemia by decreasing myocardial oxygen demand and should be continued perioperatively in CAD and heart failure patients. Sudden interruption of β-blocker has been associated with increased morbidity and mortality in CAD patients. In patients with known ischemic heart disease or patients with multiple risk factors undergoing high-risk surgery, it may be reasonable to begin β-blockers before surgery keeping in mind the adverse events such as stroke and decompensated heart failure.

Statins. Patients already on statins can continue to take them in the perioperative period. Patients with coronary artery disease, diabetes mellitus, peripheral artery disease, or chronic kidney disease and patients scheduled for major vascular surgery should be started on statins as early as possible.

Angiotensin-Converting Enzyme Inhibitors (ACEIs) and Angiotensin Receptor Blockers (ARBs). In patients with recent heart failure or uncontrolled hypertension, ACEIs or ARBs should be continued. For patients undergoing noncardiac surgery with well-controlled blood pressure, ACEIs or ARBs can be held 24 hours before surgery due to the risk for hypotension and should be started postoperatively as soon as possible.

Antiplatelets. Dual antiplatelet therapy should be interrupted in CAD patients within 30 days of bare metal stent placement and 6 months of drug-eluting stent placement. In emergent conditions, aspirin should be continued perioperatively with interruption of second antiplatelet medication for shortest duration. Patients undergoing carotid endarterectomy should have their aspirin continued unless the risk of major bleeding outweighs the benefits.

Key Points

- Asymptomatic patients with CAD can be evaluated clinically and do not require cardiac testing.
- Risk of MACE can be evaluated before noncardiac surgery by using RCRI scoring.
- Sudden interruption of CAD and heart failure medications should be avoided perioperatively.

CASE 7

Management of Cardiac Amyloidosis

A 42-year-old woman presented to the emergency department (ED) with complaint of progressive shortness of breath for 2 weeks. The symptoms were associated with leg swelling and fatigue. Her exercise tolerance was reduced from 5 blocks to 1 block. She denied fever, chest pain, palpitations, cough, and dizziness. Her medical history included diabetes mellitus, hyperlipidemia, and carpel tunnel syndrome. Medications included metformin, sitagliptin, and pravastatin. Family history included a sister who died due to heart failure at a young age. The patient denied any toxic habits. In the ED, her vital signs were stable. Physical examination revealed crackles in the lungs bilaterally, elevated jugular venous distention, and bilateral pitting pedal edema. Her ECG showed normal sinus rhythm with low-voltage QRS complex (see Figure 9.7.1). Chest x-ray showed interstitial pulmonary edema. Laboratory data revealed normal cell count, electrolytes, creatinine, thyroid function, and liver function tests. Pro-B-type natriuretic peptide and troponin levels were elevated. The patient received intravenous furosemide and was transferred to the telemetry floor for further monitoring. On the floor, echocardiography showed normal left ventricle ejection fraction, severe concentric left ventricular hypertrophy (LVH), thickened right and left atria, severely reduced longitudinal function of left ventricle, and elevated right ventricle systolic pressure (50 mm Hg). How would you further manage this case?

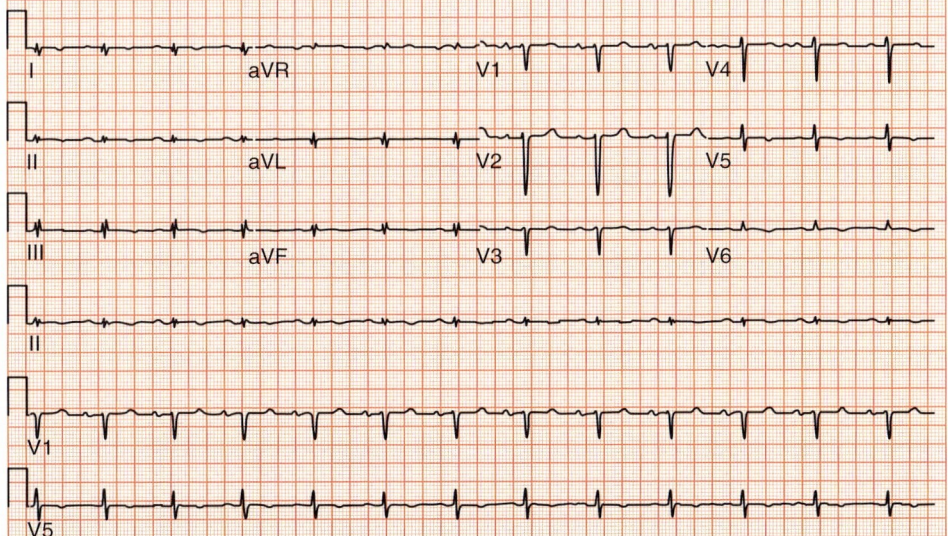

Figure 9.7.1 ECG showed normal sinus rhythm with low voltage QRS complex.

Case Review

This case describes a patient with characteristic symptoms of acute heart failure exacerbation. It is important to evaluate the etiology of heart failure in newly diagnosed cases. Evaluation for coronary artery disease is helpful, but other rare causes should also be considered, especially in patients with low cardiovascular risk factors. The characteristic ECG and echocardiographic finding in this case direct toward underlying cardiac amyloidosis as a cause of heart failure. Carpel tunnel syndrome is another associated finding. Further workup, including protein electrophoresis/immunofixation (urine/serum), free light chain measurement, technetium-99m pyrophosphate (PYP) scan, and biopsy, can be performed.

Case Discussion

Cardiac amyloidosis is an underrecognized cause of heart failure with preserved ejection fraction. It is also associated with low flow aortic stenosis. Its subtypes include the following:

- AL or primary amyloidosis (most common): Monoclonal light chains; produced in bone marrow; multiorgan involvement; cardiac has worse prognosis.
- Transthyretin (TTR): Wild or senile: mutant *TTR* >100 mutations; familial: affects heart, central nervous system; produced in liver.
- Secondary amyloidosis: Less common; associated with chronic inflammation.
- Isolated atrial amyloidosis: Common finding at autopsy.

Clinical Symptoms

Symptoms include angina in the setting of a normal coronary angiography, family history of heart failure, new-onset diabetes in elderly, proteinuria/malabsorption, bilateral carpel tunnel syndrome, lumbar spinal stenosis (multiple surgeries), macroglossia, periorbital purpura (specific in AL, infrequent), syncope or near-syncope (exertional), and cardiac thrombus.

Management

Cardiac amyloidosis is diagnosed by history and physical examination. Characteristic ECG findings include low voltage, pseudo-infarct pattern (Q waves without myocardial infarction), arrhythmia, and conduction disease. Echocardiogram can be used for both prognosis and supportive diagnosis. Typical echocardiogram findings include biatrial enlargement, LVH, right ventricular hypertrophy with pericardial effusion, speckled appearance, and strain imaging with apical sparing ("cherry on top pattern").

Although cardiac biopsy remains the gold standard for diagnosis, recently, it has been established that the ATTR variant can be reliably diagnosed in the absence of histology provided that all of the following criteria are met:

- Heart failure with an echocardiogram or cardiac magnetic resonance imaging that is consistent with or suggestive of amyloidosis
- Grade 2 or 3 cardiac uptake on a bone scan, using either 2,3-dicarboxypropane-1,1-diphosphonate (DPD) or PYP.
- Absence of a detectable monoclonal protein despite serum and urine immunofixation and serum light chains

Treatment includes management of heart failure symptoms with loop diuretics. β-Blockers and angiotensin-converting enzyme inhibitors are often not tolerated due to hypotension. Calcium channel blockers are relatively contraindicated in amyloid cardiomyopathy due to their negative ionotropic effect.

The main treatment option in patients with AL amyloidosis is chemotherapy. Bortezomib-based regimens are first-line therapy. Other options include high-dose melphalan with autologous hematopoietic stem-cell transplantation (HCT). For ATTR cardiomyopathy, tafamidis is recommended. Patisiran is an anti-TTR small interfering ribonucleic acid (siRNA) recently approved for ATTR cardiomyopathy.

Anticoagulation is recommended in patients with amyloid cardiomyopathy with atrial fibrillation or an embolic event. Prophylactic implantable cardioverter-defibrillators have been suggested to reduce the risk of sudden cardiac death.

Key Points

- Amyloid cardiomyopathy presents most commonly with unexplained heart failure symptoms.
- Diagnostic and treatment require a multidisciplinary approach.
- Prognosis is poor and correlates with the extent of the cardiac dysfunction.

CASE 8

Management of Anticoagulation in a Prosthetic Valve

A 45-year-old man with a history of mechanical mitral valve and chronic kidney disease was referred to the emergency department (ED) by his primary care physician (PCP) for management of a subtherapeutic international normalized ratio (INR). He missed a few of his warfarin doses and went to his PCP's office for follow-up, where his INR was found to be 1.5. In the ED, his vital signs were stable, and the only physical examination finding was a click at the mitral area. His creatinine was 2.5 mg/dL. He was transferred to the telemetry floor for further management. How would you treat this case?

Case Review

This case describes the management of anticoagulation in the setting of a prosthetic valve. Bridging anticoagulation with unfractionated or fractionated heparin is required to manage subtherapeutic INR in prosthetic valve patients. INR should be targeted between 2.5 and 3.5.

Case Discussion

Lifelong oral anticoagulation with warfarin is recommended for all patients with a mechanical prosthetic and those with bioprostheses with other indications for anticoagulation. The target INR is 2.5 for a mechanical aortic valve and 3 for a mechanical mitral valve. The addition of aspirin is recommended in all cases.

Bridging anticoagulation can be administered in the form of low-molecular-weight heparin (LMWH) or unfractionated heparin based on patient's comorbidities and risk factors. Usually LMWH is a convenient option for administration and has no requirement for monitoring. It should be avoided in patients with chronic kidney disease (creatinine >1.5 mg/dL) and obese patients (weight >120 kg). Unfractionated heparin is an option in patients with contraindications for LMWH unless heparin-induced thrombocytopenia is suspected.

Key Points

- Lifelong anticoagulation with warfarin is recommended in patients with a mechanical prosthetic valve.
- Aspirin should be continued in all cases.
- Target INR is 2.5 to 3.5.

CASE 9

Management of Pulmonary Regurgitation

A 58-year-old man was admitted to telemetry floor with complaints of abdominal discomfort and heaviness in his legs that had worsened in the past few weeks. He also complained of chronic cough and chest discomfort on exertion for the past 1 year. Except for a motor vehicle accident 7 years ago, he did not have any other medical history. The patient was a current chronic smoker, who smoked 1 pack per day for the past 30 years. He did not complain of any other symptoms. He worked in a shipyard for the past 25 years. Vital signs were noted as heart rate of 87 bpm, respiratory rate of 22 breaths/min, temperature of 97.4°F, and blood pressure of 148/100 mm Hg. On physical examination, the patient was thin built and found to have bilateral coarse rhonchi in the lungs. Cardiac examination revealed S_1, S_2, and a 2/6 diastolic murmur over the left second intercostal space. The patient was also found to have a positive hepatojugular reflex and bilateral pitting edema. How would you manage this case?

Case Review

This case describes a patient who presented with signs of right heart failure. The patient had been working in a shipyard industry for many years. He also had bilateral coarse crepitations, which were likely due to exposure to asbestos at his workplace, causing interstitial lung disease. Over time, interstitial lung disease can worsen and lead to pulmonary hypertension and fibrosis. This ultimately leads to pulmonary regurgitation and right ventricular failure, as in this patient.

Case Discussion

Patients with pulmonary hypertension or left heart failure leading to right heart failure can develop pulmonary regurgitation. Pulmonary regurgitation can be physiologic or pathologic. Causes include infective endocarditis, rheumatic heart disease, carcinoid disease, and congenital and iatrogenic causes. Pulmonary regurgitation causes backflow of blood into the right ventricle, initially causing right ventricular hypertrophy and later causing dilation and failure. Initially, patients are usually asymptomatic. When right heart failure sets in, these patients develop symptoms.

Clinical Symptoms

Symptoms include decreased exercise tolerance, dizziness, syncope, palpitations, fatigue, and abdominal discomfort. Examination findings include diastolic murmur, which is best heard over the left second intercostal space. Other findings include jugular venous distension, tender hepatomegaly, ascites, and pedal edema.

Management

Two-dimensional echocardiography with Doppler is the diagnostic test of choice for valvular diseases and evaluation of right ventricular function. ECG can sometimes reveal right ventricular enlargement and arrhythmias. Chest x-ray can sometimes reveal right ventricular enlargement and prominence of pulmonary trunk. Cardiac catheterization is helpful if patients have pulmonary hypertension. Other tests such CT and cardiac MRI can be used but in selected patients.

Asymptomatic patients and patients with no signs of right ventricular failure do not need any treatment. Treating the underlying cause is important. In patients with right heart failure, treatment includes use of angiotensin-converting enzyme inhibitors, β-blockers, and diuretics.

Surgery is recommended in patients with severe pulmonary regurgitation with symptoms.

Key Point

- Patient with pulmonary regurgitation need to be evaluated for underlying causes of the pulmonary regurgitation because isolated pulmonary regurgitation is rare.

CASE 10

Management of Mitral Valve Prolapse

A 38-year-old woman was admitted to the telemetry unit for evaluation of palpitations that started 2 days ago. The palpitations occurred intermittently without any association with anxiety. She recently migrated from South America 3 months ago. She denied chest pain, shortness of breath, and dizziness. Her medical history included history of myomectomy 2 years ago for fibroid uterus. No significant social or family history was noted. Her vitals were stable. Initial ECG and telemetry recording showed normal sinus rhythm with no arrhythmic events observed. Physical examination revealed long arms with increased flexibility of joints. Her lung examination was unremarkable. Cardiac auscultation revealed a grade 2/6 late systolic murmur and mid-systolic click. Further examination by auscultation revealed a decrease in murmur intensity on squatting, with the murmur returning to grade 2/6 on standing. Laboratory data, including thyroid panel and drug screen, were normal. Echocardiography showed normal ejection fraction and normal valve functions except for prolapse of the mitral valve. How would you manage this echocardiographic finding?

Case Review

This otherwise healthy patient with no symptoms was found to have an incidental finding of a cardiac murmur on auscultation. The murmur in this case is typically described as a late systolic murmur with a click classically seen in mitral valve prolapse (MVP). Additional clues to the diagnosis are her physical examination findings of long arms and increased joint flexibility. MVP can occur as an isolated finding or as a part of a syndrome, which in this case is likely Marfan syndrome. Most patients are asymptomatic, although some present with cardiac symptoms such as shortness of breath, palpitations, chest pain, dizziness, and loss of consciousness. This patient is asymptomatic and does not require treatment.

Case Discussion

MVP is a condition caused by abnormal movement of 1 or both leaflets of the mitral valve into the left atrium during systole. It can occur due to abnormality of chordae, leaflets, or papillary muscles.

MVP can be classified as primary, which includes Barlow disease and fibroelastic deficiency, or secondary, which is associated with other conditions such as connective tissue disorders, congenital heart disease, and myocardial ischemia. It can also be classified as classic, which is characterized by diffuse thickening of leaflets ≥5 mm and bileaflet prolapse, or nonclassic, which is characterized by limited or no thickening of leaflets and <5 mm of segmental prolapse. Although it remains asymptomatic, MVP can progress to severe mitral regurgitation (MR).

Clinical Symptoms

Symptoms include chest pain, exercise intolerance, dizziness, loss of consciousness, palpitations, and dyspnea.

Management

Although echocardiogram provides the definitive diagnosis, presence of systolic murmur and click can give clues to the diagnosis. Detailed clinical examination can help elucidate the underlying cause associated with MVP. Asymptomatic MVP and MVP with mild MR do not require any treatment. Patients who develop moderate to severe MR require treatment.

Key Points

- MVP is mostly asymptomatic but can present with severe presentation in some patients with severe MR.
- Echocardiography can definitively diagnose MVP.
- Evaluation is required for underlying medical conditions when suspected.

10

10×10 Abnormal Electrocardiogram, Echocardiogram, and Miscellaneous Imaging

Vincent S. Prawoko • Ayyadurai Pavanalingam • Marin Nicu

CASE 1

A 30-year-old man with a history of deep vein thrombosis and pulmonary embolism came to the hospital with a complaint of left facial numbness for 5 days with associated hearing loss in the left ear and ataxia. Echocardiography was done, and the results are shown in Figure 10.1.1.

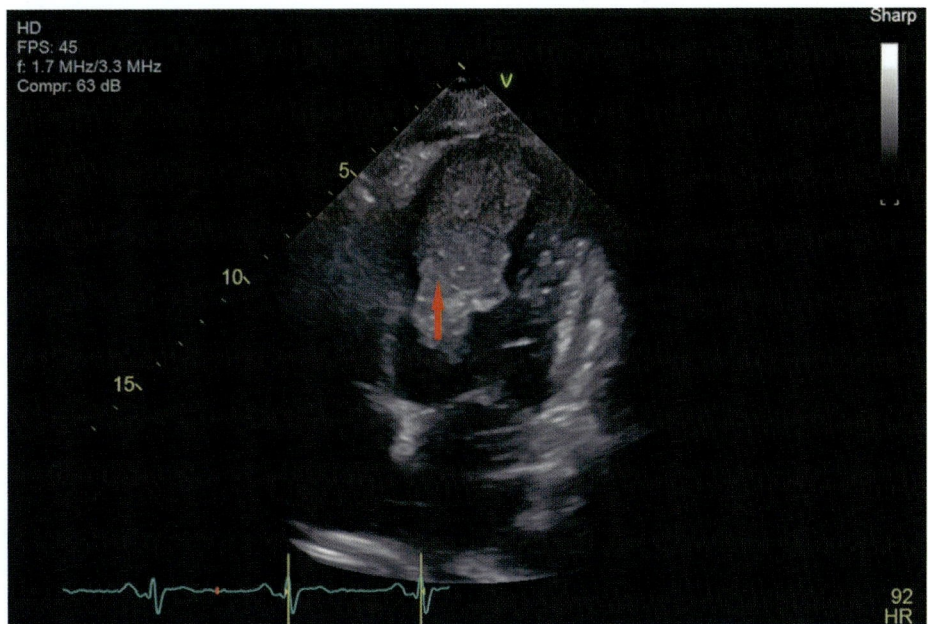

Figure 10.1.1 Echocardiography finding: Left ventricular thrombus.

Key Points

- Thrombus in the left side of the heart is very dangerous because it can lead to stroke and systemic embolism.
- Low ejection fraction, akinetic cardiac chambers, and hypercoagulable states can all lead to the occurrence of left ventricular (LV) thrombus.
- Anticoagulation with warfarin is approved for treatment of LV thrombus. Novel oral anticoagulants are not yet approved for treatment of LV thrombus.

CASE 2

A 68-year-old woman with medical history of hypertension, diabetes mellitus, and obstructive airway disease came to the hospital with complaints of chest pain. ECG did not reveal ischemic changes. Troponins were negative, and acute coronary syndrome was ruled out. Echocardiography was done, and the results are shown in Figure 10.2.1.

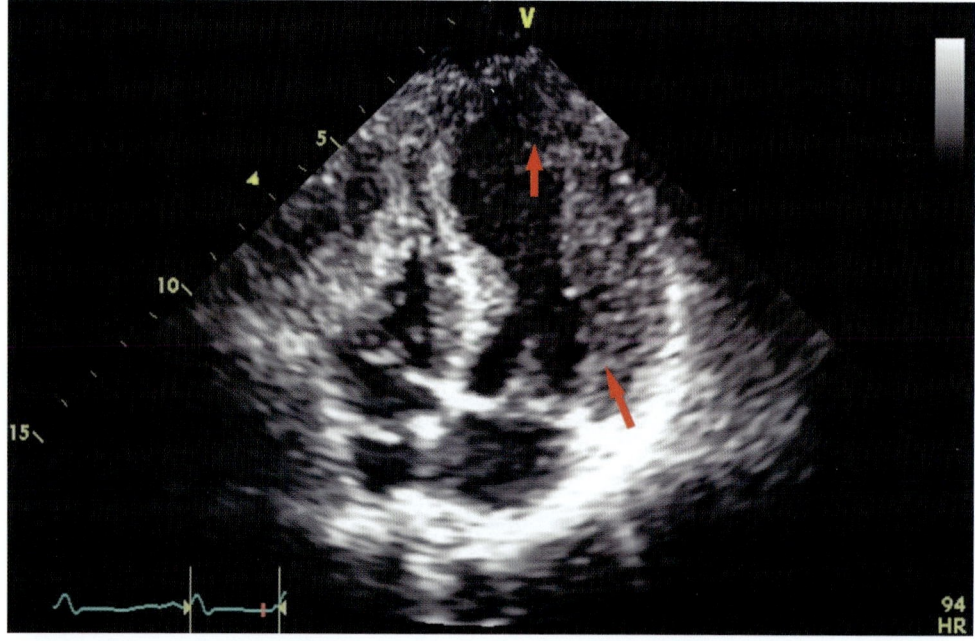

Figure 10.2.1 Echocardiography with contrast finding: Dilated ballooned apex and hyper contractile base—Classical of Takosubo cardiomyopathy.

Key Points

- Takotsubo cardiomyopathy, also called stress-induced cardiomyopathy, is characterized by regional systolic dysfunction.
- In the most common form, there is ballooning and dilatation of the apex and hypercontractility of the base.
- Takotsubo cardiomyopathy is believed to be caused by catecholamine-induced microvascular spasm.
- It is a close mimicker of acute coronary syndrome.

CASE 3

A 38-year-old man with a medical history of end-stage renal disease who is currently on hemodialysis came to the emergency department with complaints of shortness of breath. ECG showed low-voltage complexes. Echocardiography was done, and the results are shown in Figure 10.3.1.

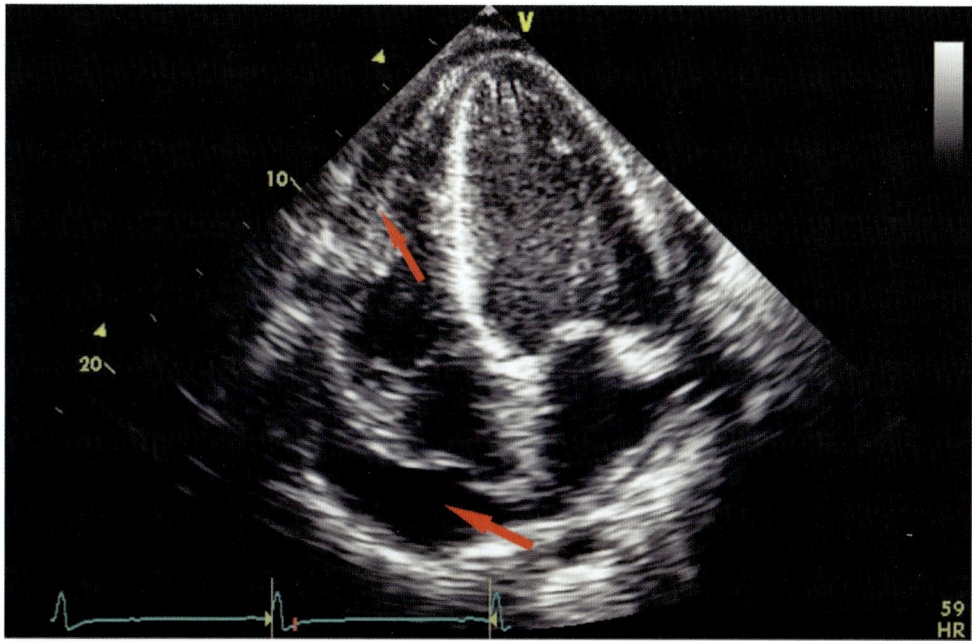

Figure 10.3.1 Echocardiogram finding: Picture showing moderate pericardial effusion, right ventricular diastolic collapse with evidence of cardiac tamponade.

Key Points

- The Beck clinical triad in cardiac tamponade includes elevated jugular venous pulsation, muffled heart sounds, and low blood pressure.
- ECG findings include low-voltage QRS complex, electrical alternans, and sinus tachycardia. However, these findings are nonspecific for cardiac tamponade.
- Echocardiography findings include right atrial systolic collapse, right ventricular diastolic collapse, inferior vena cava plethora, and increased flow variation across mitral and tricuspid valves.

CASE 4

A 53-year-old woman with medical history of hypertension, diabetes mellitus, and chronic obstructive pulmonary disease came to the emergency department with severe shortness of breath for 1 day. ECG did not show any ischemic changes. Bedside echocardiography was done, and the results are shown in Figure 10.4.1.

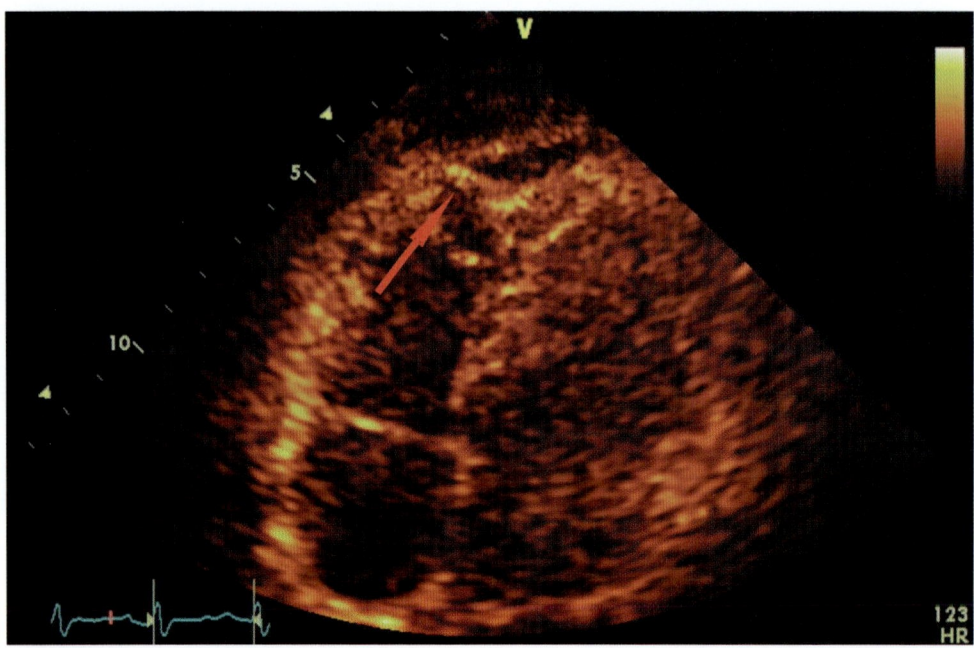

Figure 10.4.1 Echocardiography finding: Positive Mc. Connell's sign is seen in echocardiography.

Key Points

- Mc Conell's sign is characterized by akinesia of the mid free wall and hypercontractility of the apex.
- It is a highly specific finding for pulmonary embolism but not as sensitive.

CASE 5

A 47-year-old woman with a medical history of hypertension, nonischemic cardiomyopathy, and status post aortic and mitral valve replacement 5 years ago came to the hospital with fever and shortness of breath. Echocardiography was done, and the results are shown in Figure 10.5.1.

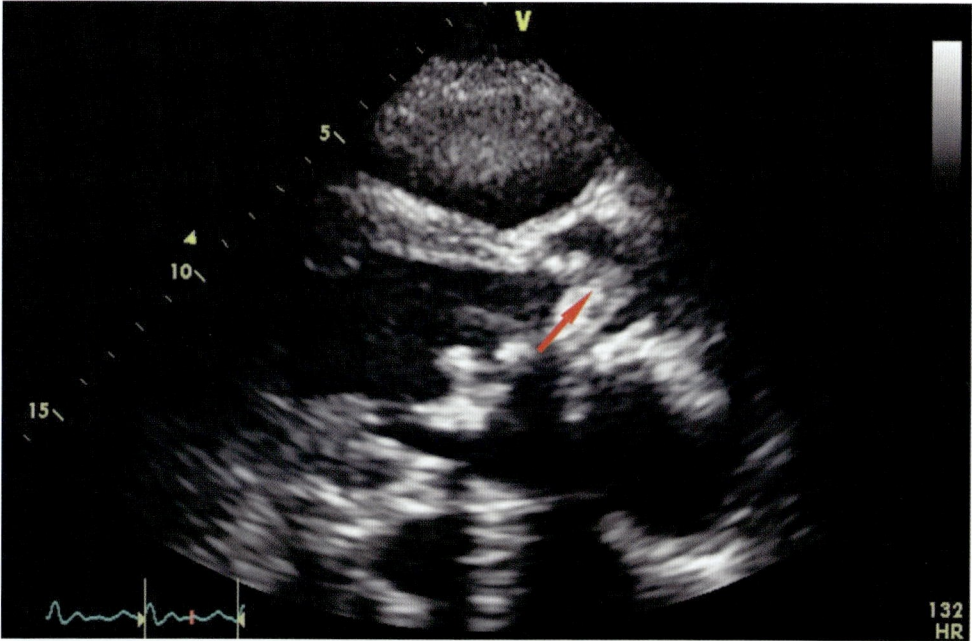

Figure 10.5.1 Echocardiography finding: Large mobile mass which may be consistent with vegetation on noncoronary cusp.

Key Points

- Patients with prosthetic heart valves are at high risk of developing infective endocarditis.
- Early treatment of infective endocarditis is important to reduce morbidity and mortality.
- Sensitivity of transthoracic echocardiography ranges from 40% to 63% for infective endocarditis and from 90% to 100% for transesophageal echocardiogrpahy.

CASE 6

A 28-year-old man with a medical history of asthma came to the hospital complaining of shortness of breath accompanied of retrosternal chest pain that was nonradiating. He rated the pain as 8/10 and indicated it was sudden in onset. He had unequal pulses in the extremities and had elevated blood pressure. CT of the chest was done, and the results are shown in Figures 10.6.1a-10.6.1b.

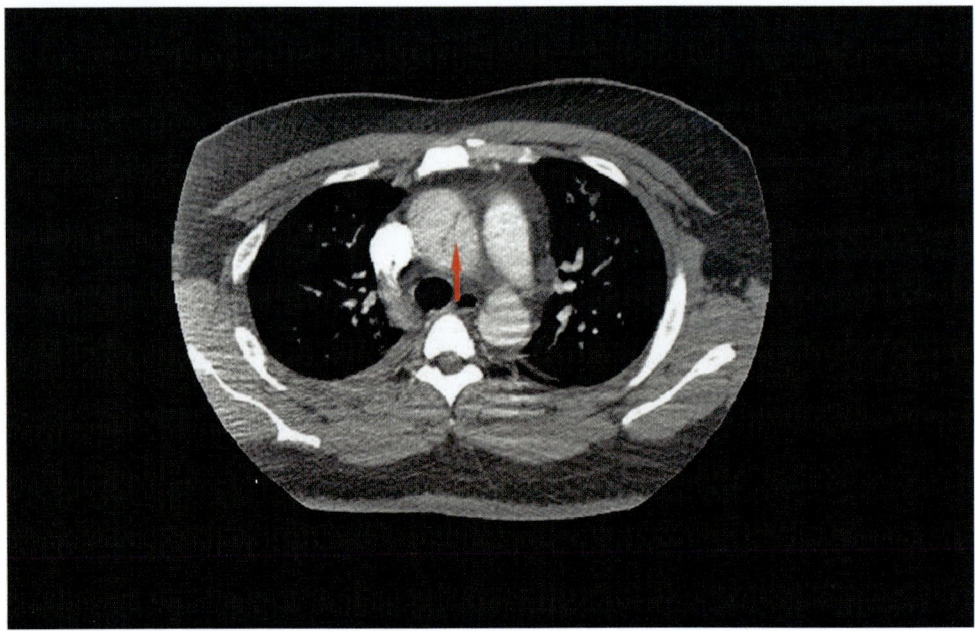

Figure 10.6.1a CT chest findings: Intimal flap is visible involving the ascending and proximal descending thoracic aorta consistent with a Stanford type A dissection.

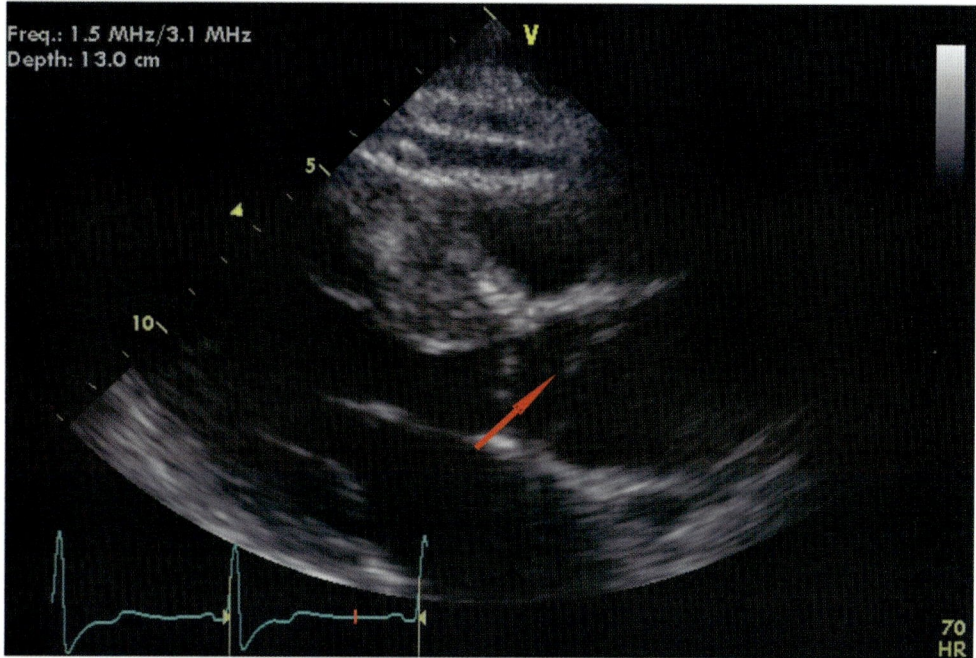

Figure 10.6.1b Echocardiogram findings: Aortic dissection flap in ascending aorta.

Key Points

- In the CT scan, an intimal flap is seen separating a false lumen from a true lumen.
- Sensitivity of transesophageal echocardiography (TEE) is as high as 98%, whereas specificity of TEE is 63% to 96%.
- CT scan has a sensitivity of 83% to 95% and a specificity of 87% to 100% for the diagnosis of acute aortic dissection.

CASE 7

An 87-year-old woman was brought to the emergency department after she passed out at home. She had a device placed for the syncope. Identify the device in the chest x-ray in Figure 10.7.1.

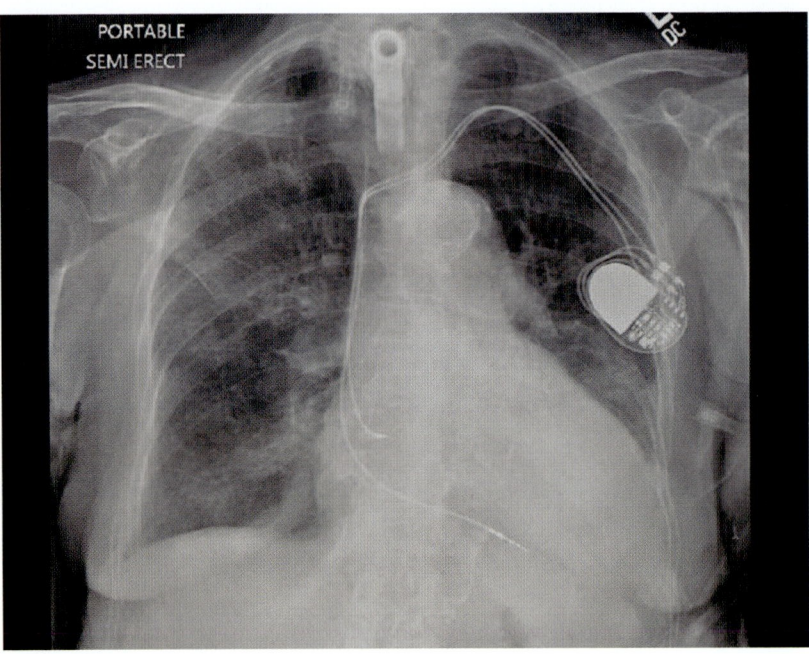

Figure 10.7.1 X-ray finding: The above patient has dual chamber pacemaker with 2 leads with one in the right atrium and one in the right ventricle.

Key Points

- Pacemakers consist of 2 components—a pulse generator and leads.
- Pacemakers are most commonly placed in the prepectoral position and are connected to 1 or more endocardial leads transvenously.
- In most pacemakers, leads are located in the endocardium, whereas in others, leads are located in the epicardium.

CASE 8

A 45-year-old patient with a medical history of cardiomyopathy and ejection fraction of 20% has come to the clinic for follow-up. Identify the device shown in Figure 10.8.1.

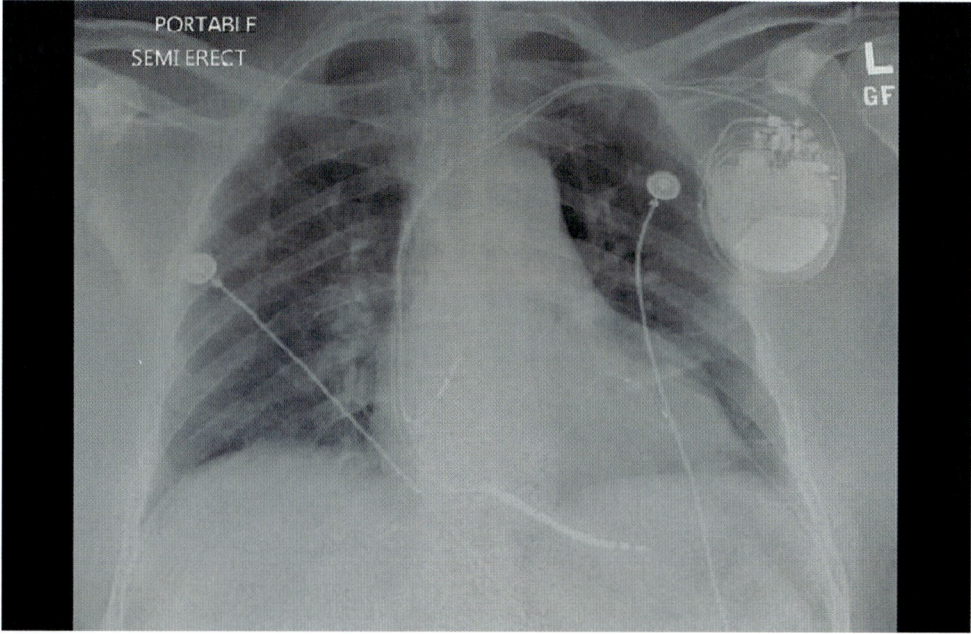

Figure 10.8.1 X-ray finding: The above device is biventricular ICD (implantable cardioverter defibrillator). The patient has a lead in right atrium, one lead in right ventricle and one in the coronary sinus for pacing the left ventricle.

Key Points

- An implantable cardioverter-defibrillator (ICD) has leads with shocking coils and a generator.
- Pacemakers do not have shocking coils.
- Shocking coils appear as thickened radiopaque structures on the leads.
- Shocking coils can be present in the right ventricular portion of the lead or in the superior vena cava portion of the lead.
- Shocking coils deliver high-energy current for defibrillation.
- Pacemakers do not have shocking coils and hence cannot shock.
- Subcutaneous ICDs have the generator and lead implanted in the subcutaneous plane.
- Pacemakers can perform pacing alone.
- ICDs can perform pacing, deliver shocks, and perform antitachycardia pacing.

CASE 9

A 56-year-old male patient with the history of hypertension, schizophrenia, and hypothyroidism presented to emergency department with shortness of breath and chest pain. ECG done in the emergency department showed ST elevations in leads V_2 to V_5. He was taken to the cardiac catheterization lab and angiogram showed the following (see Figures 10.9.1a-10.9.1c).

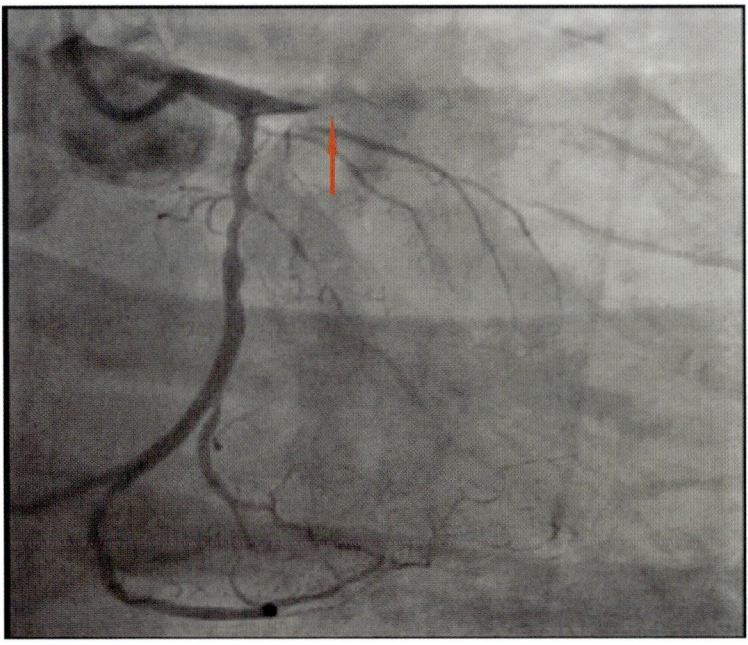

Figure 10.9.1a Coronary angiogram showing proximal left anterior descending artery occlusion.

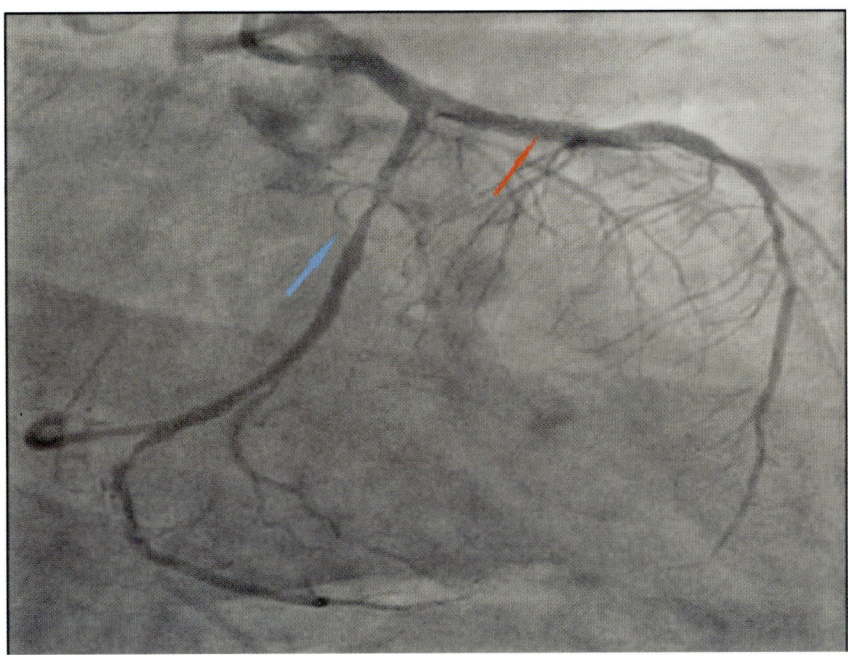

Figure 10.9.1b Coronary angiogram post PCI showing restoration of flow (red arrow). It also shows left circumflex artery (blue arrow).

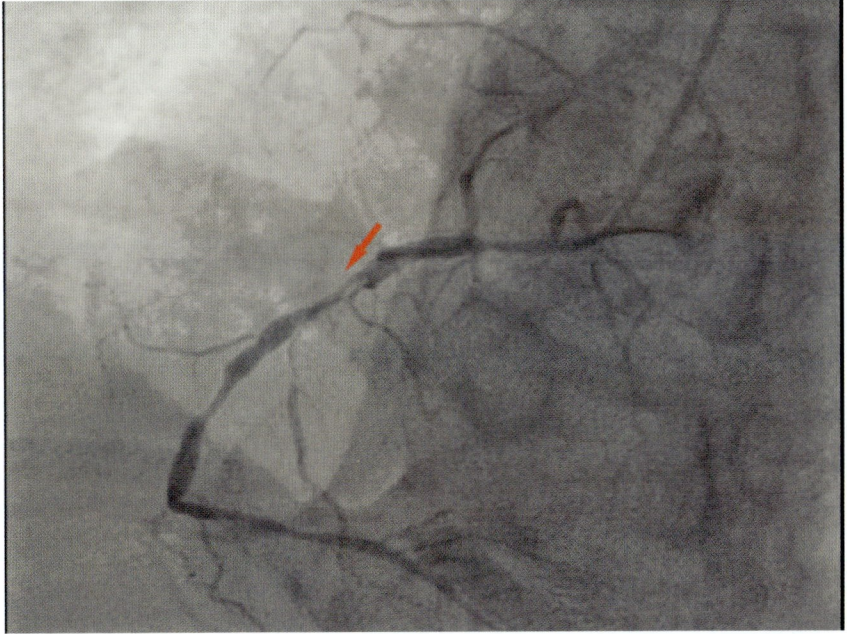

Figure 10.9.1c Right coronary artery with 70% occlusion in proximal and mid RCA.

Key Points

- ST-segment elevation myocardial infarction (STEMI) presents with ST-segment elevation on ECG and is due to acute plaque rupture, which causes complete occlusion of the coronary artery.
- Primary percutaneous coronary intervention (PCI) improves mortality in STEMI.
- Primary PCI is superior to thrombolytics for STEMI management.

CASE 10

A 62-year-old man with a medical history of hypertension, diabetes mellitus, and hyperlipidemia came to the emergency department with shortness of breath. The patient was found to have new-onset atrial fibrillation. He was planned for cardioversion. He had a transesophageal echocardiography (TEE), which showed the following results. (Figures 10.10.1a-10.10.1b).

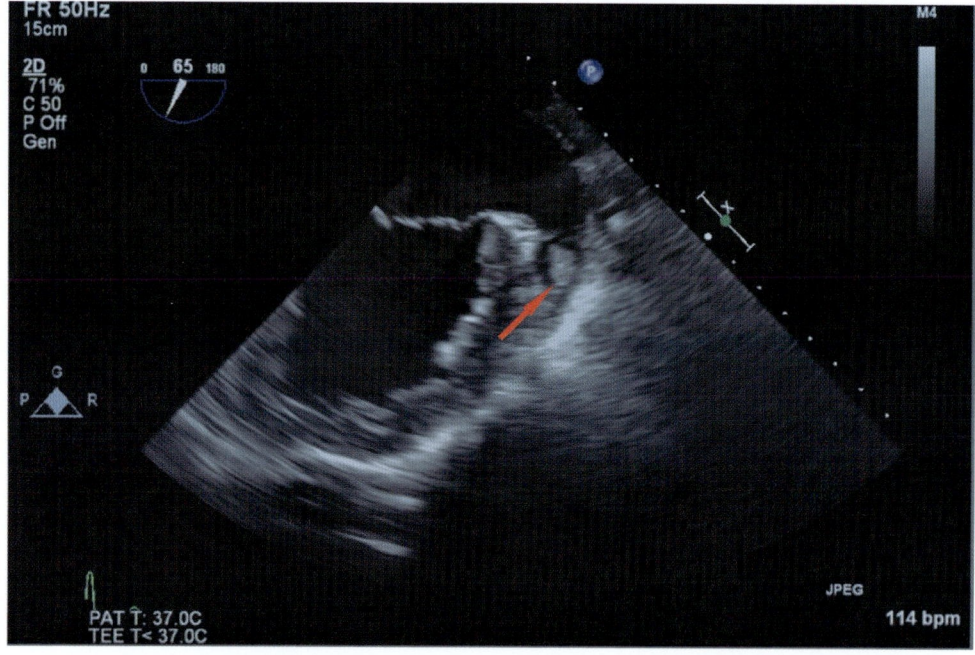

Figure 10.10.1a TEE findings: Large 0.90 × 1.25 cm sized pedunculated mobile thrombus was visualized in left atrial appendage.

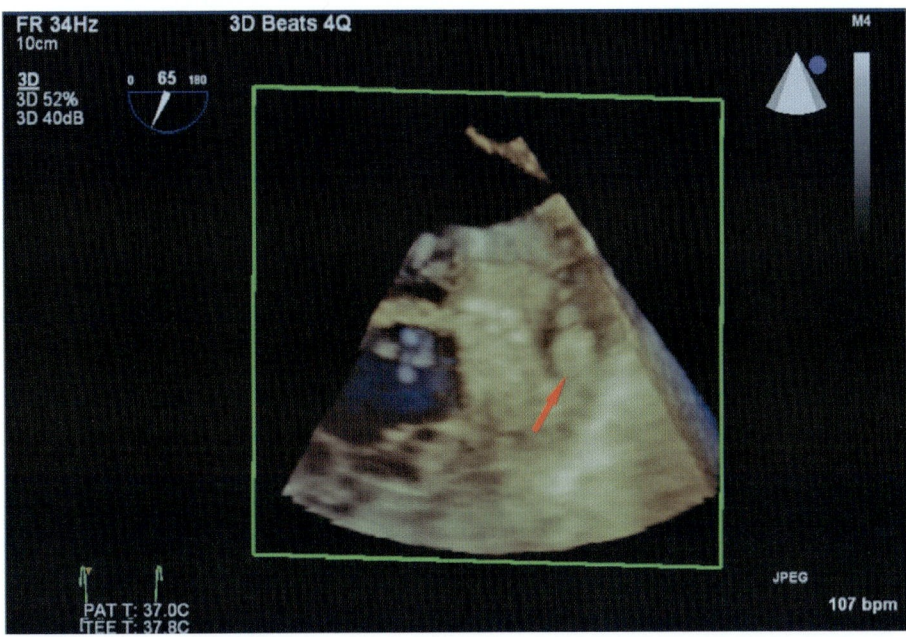

Figure 10.10.1b   TEE findings: Large 0.90 × 1.25 cm sized pedunculated mobile thrombus was visualized in left atrial appendage.

Key Points

- Left atrial appendage thrombus is an independent predictor of thromboembolic risk and is associated with increased risk of stroke.
- Treatment includes anticoagulation with warfarin.
- Novel oral anticoagulants have not been approved for treatment of left atrial appendage thrombus.

CASE 11

A 50-year-old woman presented to the hospital with syncope after shopping. She did not have chest pain. She had shortness of breath on exertion for the past 1 year, and her exercise tolerance was decreasing. Echocardiography was done, and it showed the following results. (Figure 10.11.1).

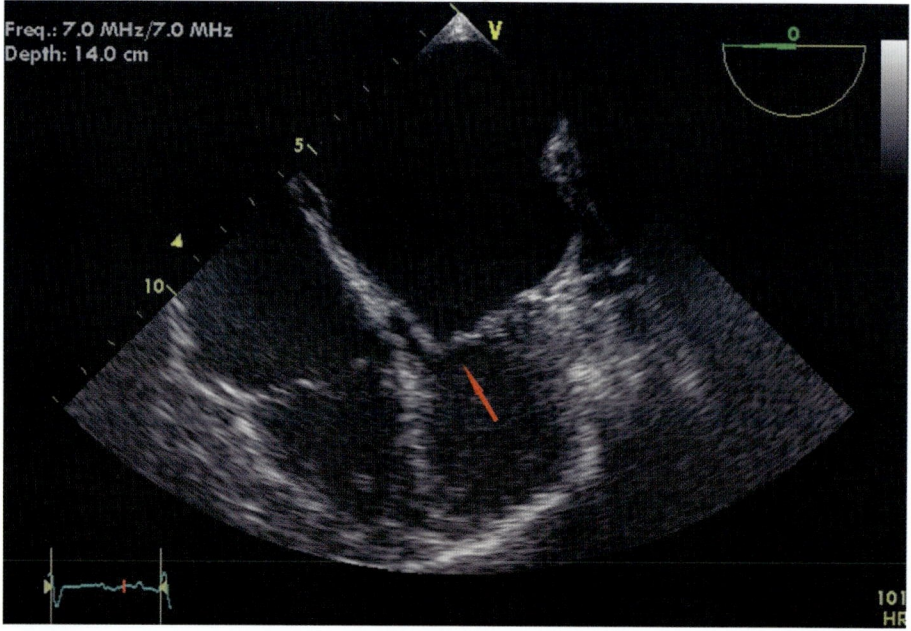

Figure 10.11.1 Echocardiography findings: Severe mitral stenosis.

Key Points

- Mitral stenosis is the most common valvular heart disease in the developing world.
- Rheumatic heart disease is the most common cause of mitral stenosis worldwide.
- Treatment of mitral stenosis includes mitral valvotomy or mitral valve replacement.

CASE 12

A 45-year-old woman presented with palpitations that started 1 hour ago. She also reported chest discomfort during this event. ECG is shown in Figure 10.12.1.

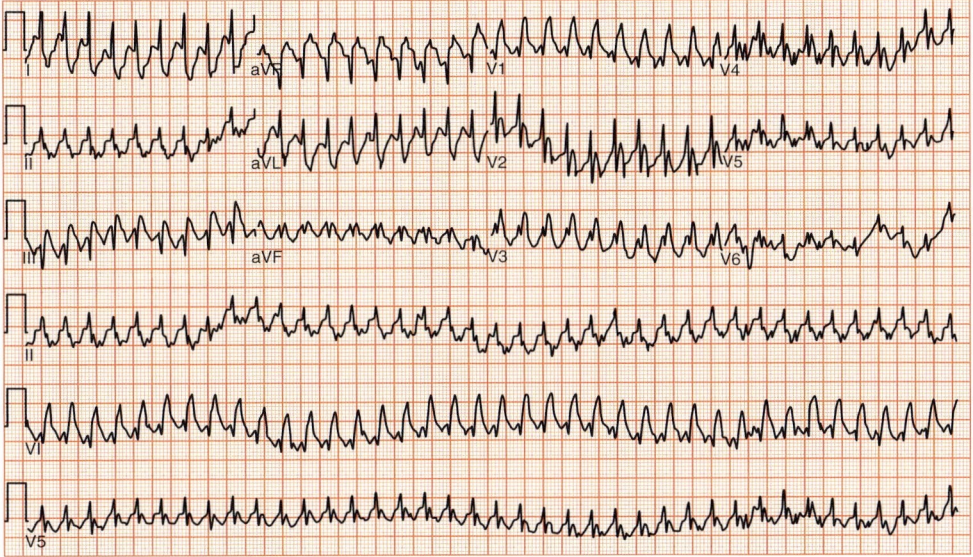

Figure 10.12.1 Finding: This ECG shows that she has supraventricular tachycardia (SVT) with the rate of 250 beats/minute. This patient has long RP tachycardia and adenosine will help in definite diagnosis.

Key Points

- Supraventricular tachycardia (SVT) includes all tachycardias that originate above the ventricles.
- According to American Heart Association, SVTs include inappropriate sinus tachycardia, atrial tachycardia (AT; including focal and multifocal AT), macro-reentrant AT (including typical atrial flutter), junctional tachycardia, atrioventricular nodal reentry tachycardia, and various forms of accessory pathway–mediated reentrant tachycardias.

CASE 13

A 37-year-old man presented to emergency department complaining of worsening palpitations and dizziness for 1 day. He said that the palpitations are intermittent and started 1 week ago. ECG showed the following results. (Figure 10.13.1).

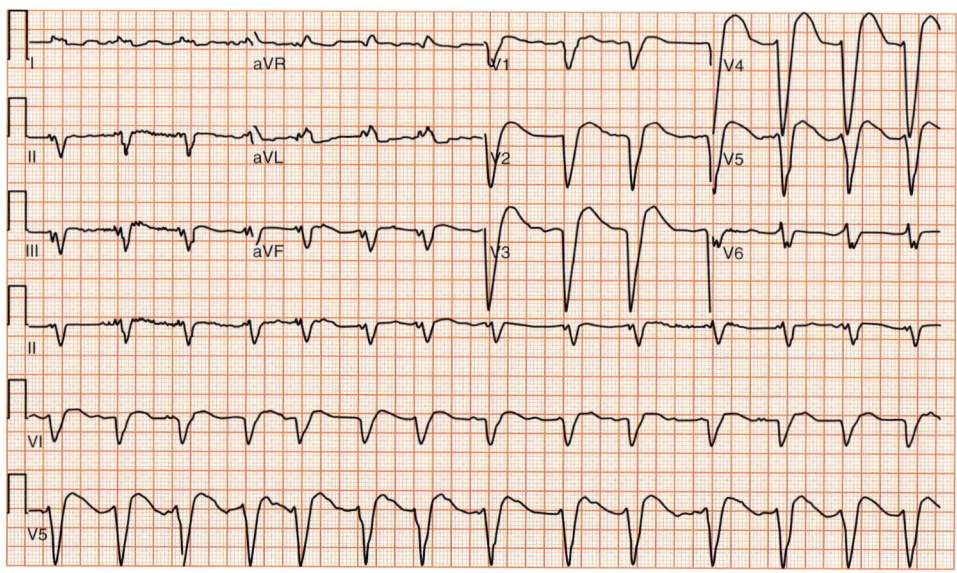

Figure 10.13.1 Finding: This ECG shows atrial fibrillation with intra-ventricular block.

Key Points

- Atrial fibrillation is diagnosed when an irregularly irregular narrow complex rhythm is found with no P wave seen in front of the QRS complexes.
- Fibrillary waves can sometimes be present.

CASE 14

A 57-year-old woman presented with right-sided weakness and was found to have had an acute stroke. She was noted to be tachycardic, and her pulse was irregular. Her ECG showed the following results. (Figure 10.14.1).

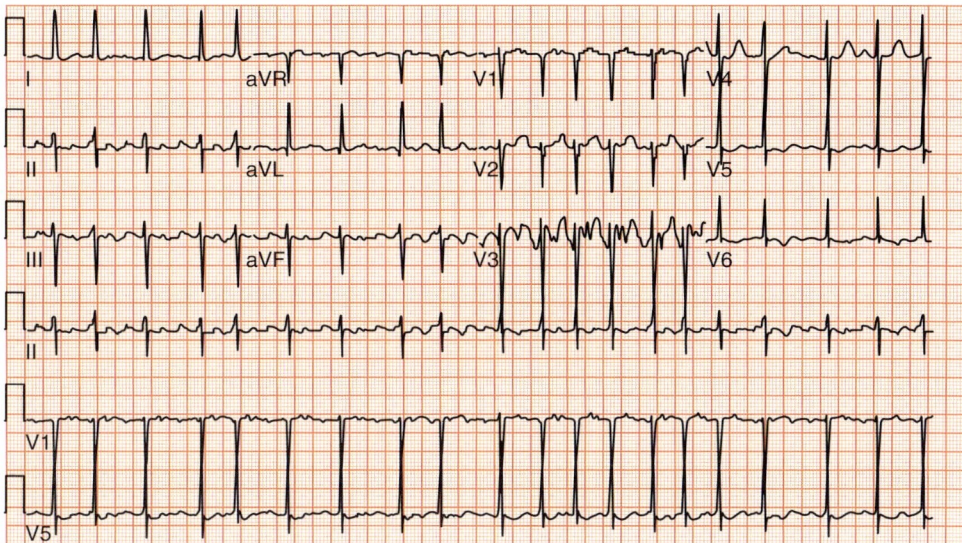

Figure 10.14.1   Finding: This ECG shows atrial flutter with variable block with ventricular rate of 120/minute. R-R interval is variable and sawtooth flutter waves are seen in the ECG.

Key Points

- Atrial flutter can be seen on ECG as a sawtooth pattern of the P wave. The ratio of the flutter wave to QRS may be fixed such as 1:1, 2:1, 3:1, or more, but it also may vary.
- Atrial flutter is classified as cavotricuspid isthmus (CTI)-dependent flutter or CTI-independent flutter. CTI-dependent flutter uses the macro-reentrant circuit in the CTI area in the right atrium.
- Ablation is curative for this type of atrial flutter.

CASE 15

A 40-year-old man was seen in the cardiology clinic for a routine follow-up for his hypertension. He did not have any complaints and felt fine. ECG was done and showed the following results. (Figure 10.15.1).

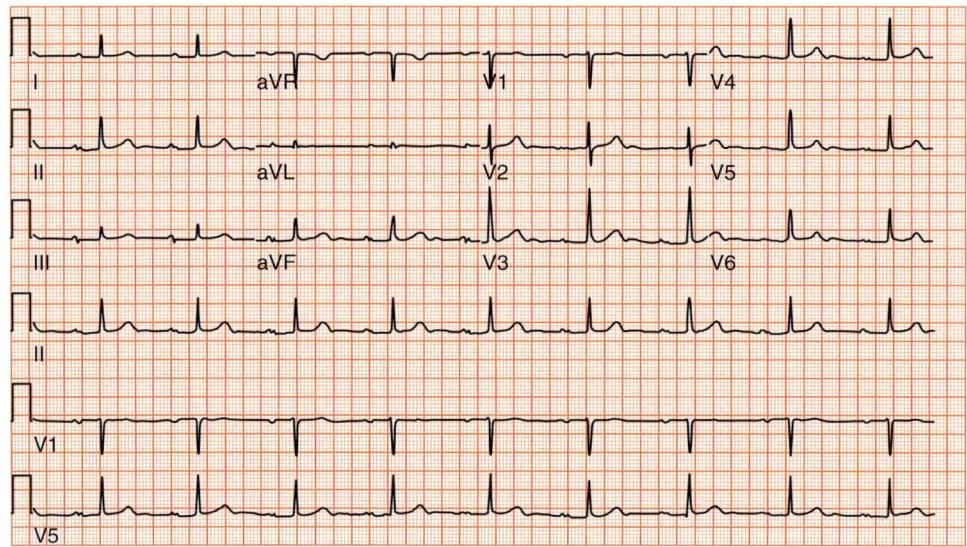

Figure 10.15.1 Findings: This ECG shows sinus rhythm with first-degree AV block.

Key Points

- First-degree atrioventricular block is diagnosed when the PR interval is lengthened to >0.20 seconds on ECG.
- In asymptomatic patients, it requires no intervention.

CASE 16

A 77-year-old woman was seen for the first time in the clinic. She said that she had long-standing hypertension and some irregularity of her heartbeats. ECG showed the following results. (Figure 10.16.1).

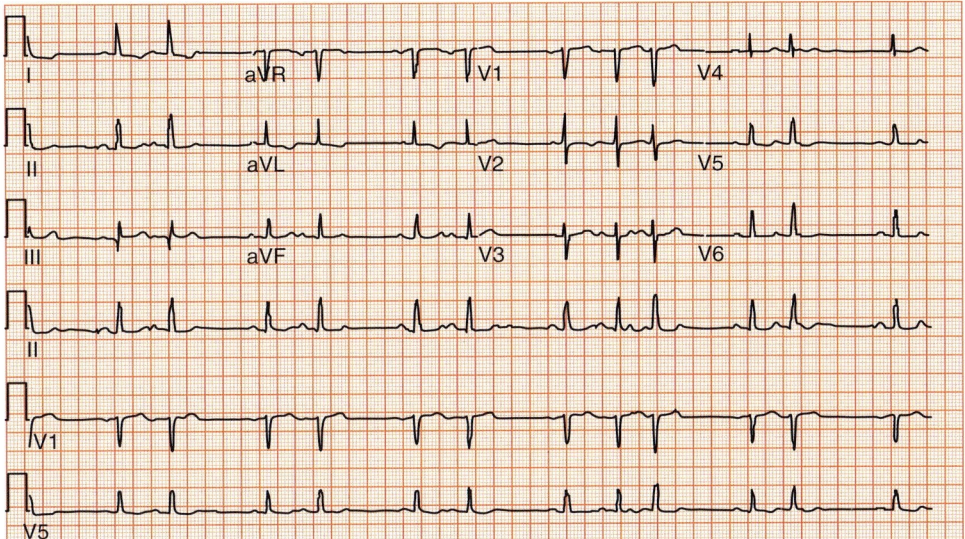

Figure 10.16.1 Findings: This ECG shows that she has AV block second degree, Mobitz type I.

Key Points

- Type I second-degree atrioventricular (AV) block can be identified by looking at the PR interval on the ECG. The PR interval in this type on AV block is progressively lengthened and followed by a blocked P wave.
- In Mobitz type I heart block, the level of the block is usually at the AV node.

CASE 17

A 76-year-old woman was brought to the emergency department by her family due to acute change in mental status. As per the family, she had also been complaining of abdominal pain for the past 2 hours. She had a medical history of diabetes mellitus, hypertension, and gastritis. ECG is shown in Figure 10.17.1.

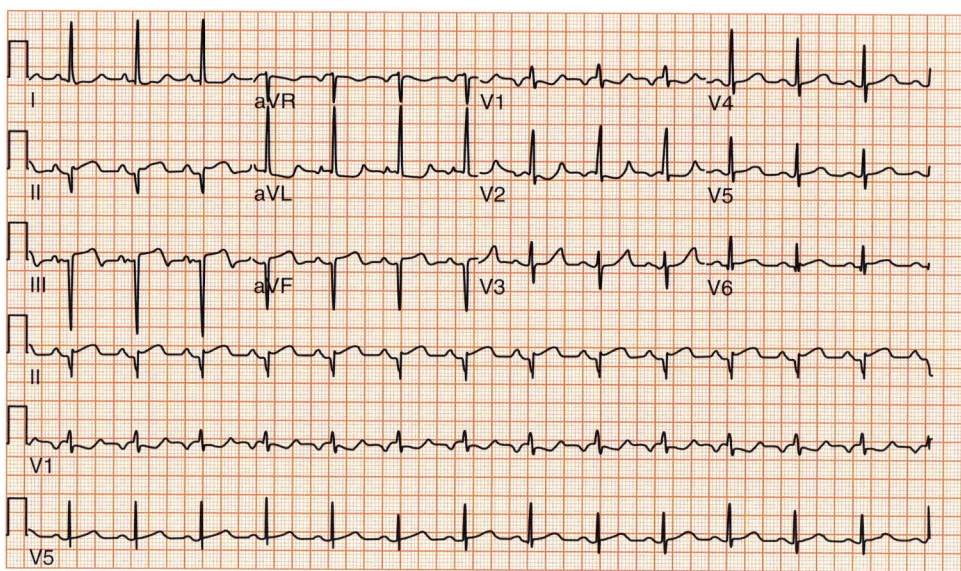

Figure 10.17.1 Findings: This ECG shows sinus rhythm with ST elevation on leads II, III, and AVF with reciprocal changes of ST depression on leads V_1 and V_2. This is consistent with inferior STEMI—with possibility of also posterior MI.

Key Points

- ST-segment elevation myocardial infarction (STEMI) is characterized by ST-segment elevation on ECG in at least 2 contiguous leads.
- In STEMI, reciprocal changes are also seen, characterized by ST-segment depression on the opposite side leads. When you see ST-segment depression on leads V_1 to V_3, a posterior lead ECG with V_7, V_8, and V_9 can be performed to diagnose posterior wall myocardial infarction (MI).
- Other findings suspicious of posterior MI are R/S ratio of >1 in V_2 and tall, broad R wave with upright T wave.

CASE 18

A 60-year-old woman came to the cardiology clinic for follow-up after pacemaker placement 1 month ago. The ECG done at this visit showed the following results. (Figure 10.18.1).

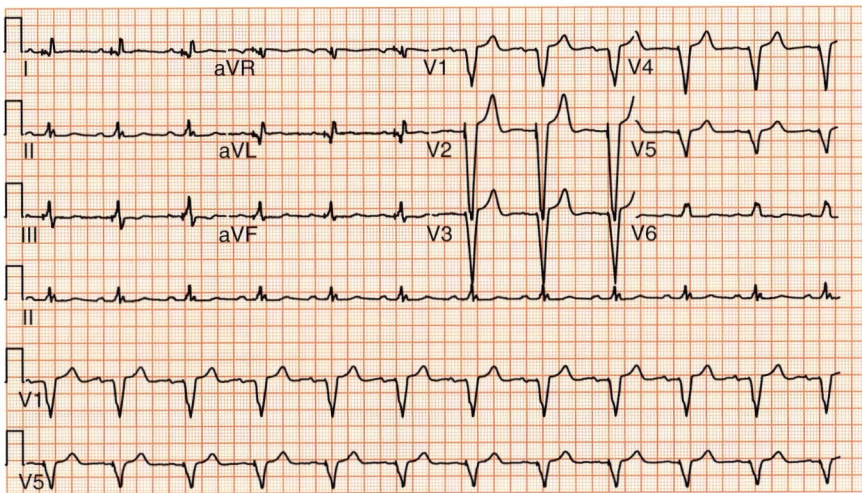

Figure 10.18.1 Findings: This ECG shows paced rhythm around 70 beats/minute. We can also see the LBBB pattern on this ECG.

Key Points

- Paced rhythm can be identified by looking at the spike before P wave or QRS complex.
- Left bundle branch block pattern on a paced rhythm indicates that the pacing starts from the right ventricle.

CASE 19

A 55-year-old man was seen in the cardiology clinic for a routine follow-up. He had a pacemaker placed a few years ago due to symptomatic bradycardia. He denied any symptoms and was in a good condition. ECG showed the following results. (Figure 10.19.1).

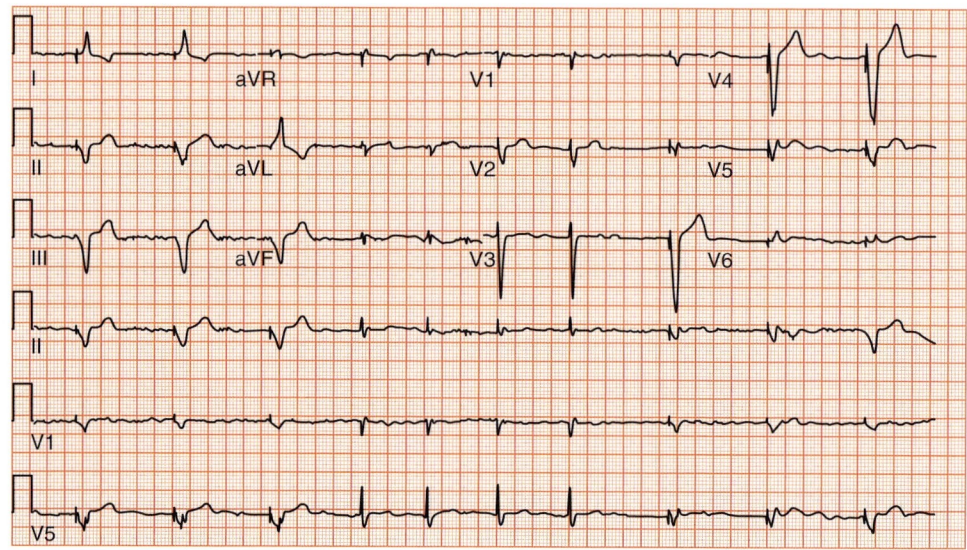

Figure 10.19.1 Findings: This ECG shows ventricular demand pacing.

Key Point

- Ventricular demand pacing can be seen by looking at intermittent pacing rhythm on ECG. This means that the pacemaker paces the heart when it drops below the threshold that was set on the device.

CASE 20

A 56-year-old man suddenly collapsed during his cardiology appointment. He came in due to intermittent brief palpitations associated with dizziness for the past few days. He had a medical history of hypertension, diabetes mellitus, and heart failure with reduced ejection fraction (ejection fraction, 20%; patient had implantable cardioverter-defibrillator placed 2 years ago). ECG was immediately performed and revealed the following results. (Figure 10.20.1).

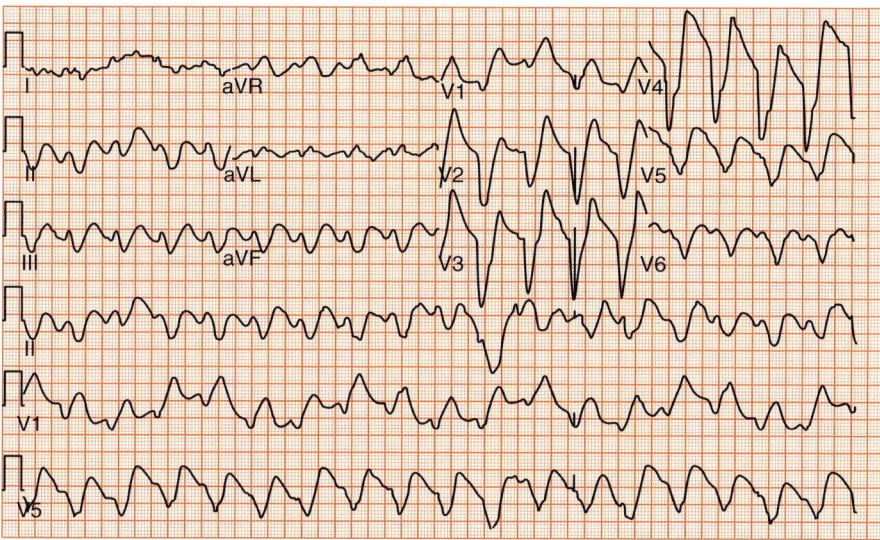

Figure 10.20.1 Findings: This ECG shows ventricular tachycardia (VT). We can also see pacemaker spike on one of the waves.

Key Points

- Ventricular tachycardia (VT) is characterized by a wide QRS complex (≥120 milliseconds) tachycardia (>100 bpm).
- Further characterization of VT includes sustained (≥30 seconds) or nonsustained and monomorphic or polymorphic.
- ECG also shows negative concordance in leads V_1 to V_6 that is highly suggestive of ventricular tachycardia.

Index

Note: Page numbers followed by *f* and *t* indicate figures and tables, respectively.

Transient ischemic attack and stroke cases (*Cont.*):
lacunar stroke, 127–128
large-vessel stroke, 113–115
migraine with brainstem aura, 121–122
transient ischemic attack, 115–117, 116*t*
vertebral artery dissection, 122–124
Transthoracic echocardiography (TTE)
constrictive pericarditis diagnosis with, 103
left ventricular ejection fraction in, 85–86
PE evaluation with, 10
Tremors, hypomagnesemia with, 154
Tricuspid regurgitation, 65–66
Tricuspid stenosis, 72–74
Tricyclic antidepressants, costochondritis treatment
with, 7
Triptans, pseudosyncope treatment with, 52
TTE. *See* Transthoracic echocardiography
Twiddler syndrome, 47

U
Unstable angina (UA), 3–4
Upper extremity peripheral arterial disease, 132–133

V
Valvular heart disease
aortic regurgitation with, 68–69
aortic stenosis with, 60–61
bicuspid aortic valve with, 66–67
coarctation of aorta with, 71–72
heart failure etiology with, 77
heart failure with preserved EF with, 82–83
mitral regurgitation with, 63–65
mitral stenosis with, 61–63
patent foramen ovale with, 59–60
pulmonary stenosis with, 70–71
tricuspid regurgitation with, 65–66
tricuspid stenosis with, 72–74

Vasodilators, angina variants treated with, 6
Venous Doppler duplex ultrasound, 10
Venous thromboembolism, chest pain with, 9
Ventricular demand pacing, 184, 184*f*
Ventricular tachycardia
ECG of, 22*f*, 23, 185, 185*f*
management of, 22–23, 22*f*
STEMI notification with, 22–23
symptoms of, 23
Vertebral artery dissection
head and neck trauma associated with, 123
management of, 122–124
Vertigo, migraine with brainstem aura with, 121
Vestibular neuronitis, peripheral vertigo caused by,
41
Vestibular schwannoma, 41
Vomiting
alcohol withdrawal syndrome with, 54
hypertensive encephalopathy with, 91–92
hyponatremia with, 150
intracerebral hemorrhage with, 119
large-vessel stroke with, 114
migraine-related syncope with, 50
resistant hypertension with, 96
sympathomimetic drug overdose with, 95

W
Wells score pretest probability, 10
Wenckebach phenomenon. *See* Mobitz type I
second-degree AV block
Wolff-Parkinson-White (WPW) syndrome, 31

X
X-ray
implantable cardioverter-defibrillator in, 171,
171*f*
pacemaker in, 170, 170*f*